The Town That Lost a TON

How one town used the
BUDDY SYSTEM to lose 3,998 POUNDS...
and how you can too!

Jane Clemen, R.D., L.D.

Dianna Kirkwood, M.A.

Bobbi Schell, P.T.

With Daniel Myerson

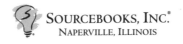
SOURCEBOOKS, INC.
NAPERVILLE, ILLINOIS

This publication is designed to provide accurate and authoritative information in regard to the subject matter covered. It is sold with the understanding that the publisher is not engaged in rendering legal, accounting, or other professional service. If legal advice or other expert assistance is required, the services of a competent professional person should be sought.—*From a Declaration of Principles Jointly Adopted by a Committee of the American Bar Association and a Committee of Publishers and Associations*

Trademarks: All brand names and product names used in this book are trademarks, reg-istered trademarks, or trade names of their respective holders. Sourcebooks, Inc., is not associated with any product or vendor in this book.

All efforts have been made to secure permissions for the recipes used within this text. If any errors have been made, we will be happy to correct them in future editions.

Published by Sourcebooks, Inc.
P.O. Box 4410, Naperville, Illinois 60567-4410
(630) 961-3900
FAX: (630) 961-2168
www.sourcebooks.com

Library of Congress Cataloging-in-Publication Data

Clemen, Jane.
 The town that lost a ton : how one town lost 3,998 pounds– and how you can too! Jane Clemen, Bobbi Schell, Dianna Kirkwood
     p. cm.
 ISBN 1-57071-746-X
1. Weight loss. 2. Weight loss–Iowa–Dyersville. I. Schell, Bobbi.
II. Kirkwood, Dianna. III. Title.
RM222.2 .C5185 2002
613.7–dc21

                                                   2001006798

Printed and bound in the United States of America
BG   10   9   8   7   6   5   4   3   2

We dedicate this book to the nearly three thousand people who have embraced Fight the Fat on their journey to a healthier life. Their spirit and enthusiasm have led us and allowed us to consider ourselves wonderful works in progress. Remarkable people have made Fight the Fat and this book reality.

Table of Contents

Preface   xi
Chapter One: Town of Dreams   1
Chapter Two: Your Own Dyersville   20
Chapter Three: The Meeting   40
Chapter Four: Stress   61
Chapter Five: Who *Is* That?   82
Chapter Six: Mid-diet Slump!   106
Chapter Seven: Glorious Food   133
Chapter Eight: Look Out, World   161
Chapter Nine: Handling Others   183
Chapter Ten: Beginning   204

Acknowledgments

Six women, Patti Bell, Nancy Dunkel, Becky Friedman, Sharon Gudenkauf, Dr. Mary O'Connell, and Ina Pape, joined us nearly five years ago and clearly told us what the community needed from their local health care provider. They generously gave wonderful ideas and hours of help. Glady Felton joined in to be the glue that held us all statistically together. The staff at Total Fitness Recreation Center with Mary, Christy, and Andrea became an integral part of the program and spurred even more ideas. Other community sponsors (especially our KDST friend Doug) and the original participants believed in us enough to jump on our bandwagon.

Through it all, the understanding, support, and trust of Jeanette Digmann, Rod Tokheim, Deb Poppe, Rusty Knight, and the staff in our Physical Rehab, Nutrition, and Community Relations Departments kept us going.

Noah Lukeman, our literary agent whom we tested at every turn, demonstrated vision, perseverance, and endless patience. He also introduced us to a treasured friend. And to our comrades in this adventure, without your organization, imagination, and spirit, this simply wouldn't have been possible.

And finally, special thanks to our editor Hillel Black for having had the vision to take on this project!

To all of you, we say thank you for believing, trusting, and caring.

Thanks to my husband Roger. Your love and support have empowered me to pursue new challenges. Thank you also to my children Curt, Dana, and Doug, for your patience and love.—Jane Clemen, Director of Nutrition for Mercy Medical Center, Dyersville, Iowa

Thank you to Tom who endlessly supports and encourages me as I chase ideas, opportunities, and adventures. And to Shona, Kory, Nickie, and Kearn, thanks for encouraging and inspiring me. I have learned so much from all of you.—Dianna Kirkwood, Director of Marketing for Mercy Medical Center, Dyersville, Iowa

To my family—Randy, Megan, Katie, and Susie—thank you for giving me the time to be the Fight the Fat cheerleader and for believing in me. To my friends—Gloria, Jan, Joan, Mary, Nancy, and Susie—I couldn't have done any of this without your love and support.—Bobbi Schell, Supervisor of Rehabilitation Outreach Services at Mercy Medical Center, Dyersville, Iowa

First and foremost, I want to thank Eliezer Krawiec and Eliyahu Vaiselberg for extraordinary help in the technical aspects of this book. They are truly remarkable and unique individuals. Special thanks to Brenda Shoshanna and Leah Kohn for their unfailing support and love. Thanks to Shana and Lisa Saposh, chefs extraordinaire, for their input. Thanks to Suzanne Plavé for her words of wisdom and to Francine Plavé for her insightful criticism.

— Daniel Myerson

Preface

"Is this heaven? No, it's Iowa!"
—From the movie *Field of Dreams*

The purpose of this book is to help people *permanently* change their lives, to permit them to fulfill their potential for health, energy, and zest for living. You will come to *love and enjoy* your new healthy lifestyle, and that is why the changes brought about by the Fight the Fat program will last. Diets don't work because they are short periods of deprivation followed by an orgy of eating—the inevitable *I'm going to make up for the suffering* reaction.

Fight the Fat works because during the ten-week program you acquire new habits! You discover new healthy foods that come to be *more* satisfying than your old favorites. You learn ways to deal with stress that are more effective than bingeing and that leave you feeling better. Fight the Fat offers you challenges, stimulation, and rewards.

What's more, an important key to success during your ten weeks of Fight the Fat is working with others. What makes all the difference is the support you get from your teammates—and the support you give them as well!

It doesn't matter whether you choose to start up a Fight the Fat team with two or two hundred members. All you need is one other person. Chapter two explains how you can get a team started at work, at home, with a friend, or with a stranger, suggesting ways you can organize a mini-team and outlining the possibilities for larger groups as well.

It also doesn't matter whether you are from Dyersville, Iowa, or New York, New York. Fight the Fat works anywhere because the program was created to deal with the *everyday needs of people.* That was the bottom line for the Fight the Fat organizers—three dedicated colleagues from Dyersville's Mercy Medical Center: Director of Nutrition Jane Clemen, Supervisor of Rehabilitation Outreach Services Bobbi Schell, and Director of Marketing Dianna Kirkwood. Working at Mercy, these women saw the suffering caused by excess weight on a daily basis. So, they got together and brainstormed, coming up with the ten-week Fight the Fat program that can be, and is, repeated with great success over and over again.

These women had no idea that the whole town of Dyersville would eventually get involved, or that the program would spread to surrounding towns and cities! But word of their success caught on, inspiring many people to join! (Currently, in Dubuque, Iowa, for example, five hundred people attend a Fight the Fat meeting every week in the shopping mall.) Jane, Bobbi, and Dianna understand that people need the help of others to deal with their weight problem; it can be just too much for them to struggle on their own.

This is what Fight the Fat is about—ordinary people who changed their lives by teaming up. Their idea was what a generation ago farmers called "To Neighbor." People helped one another and they discovered that in the process they were also helping themselves. In Dyersville, people who had been unable to motivate themselves for a lifetime suddenly found themselves standing together with their team on a huge truck scale, each wearing their team shirt, embarking on a campaign to turn their lives around. In ten short weeks, a small middle-American town made history, losing 3,998 pounds together and sparking a new concept in health and fitness.

Although it started in Iowa, a team with the Iowa spirit—and the Iowa approach—can be found with a group of big city people who walk their dogs in the same park every morning! Two coworkers can do it; two couples who meet for cards every weekend can do it, "it" being whatever part of the program fits their needs! The point is that big organizations give you mass-produced answers: Fight the Fat teams work to build up support one-to-one between teammates. It addresses the special needs that you and only you have when you struggle to become fit.

When you and your Fight the Fat partner team up—and remember, we're talking about even just two people here—you create a whole new mind-set. Different responses, different attitudes, and different reactions take place without you knowing it, at first. You are bonding with your teammate. You are taking control. The same phenomenon occurs on an athletic team: you tap into your own strength and the strength of your teammates. You strive to be the best you can be *together*.

Each one of the ten weeks in the Fight the Fat campaign has an overall theme, a special emphasis or focus:

- Week One: Getting started
- Week Two: Creating your team
- Week Three: The meeting
- Week Four: Stress
- Week Five: Exercise
- Week Six: Mid-diet slump
- Week Seven: Food!
- Week Eight: Motivation!
- Week Nine: Dealing with others
- Week Ten: Maintaining what you have achieved

Weekly Workbook

In addition, to help you on your way each chapter concludes with an interactive weekly workbook consisting of many sections to help you along.

The Bulletin Board

The bulletin board contains the wit and wisdom of a wide range of people—from Arnold Schwarzenegger on weight lifting to Grandma Moses on life! Quotations are brought together to inspire and motivate you, to give you a new way of looking at problems and challenges. Glancing at your bulletin board every day will give you an extra shot of willpower and encouragement!

Your Journal

Every week you are also given questions that will make you stop and think about the issues involved in weight loss (you can either write the answers or speak them into a tape recorder). You will do some delving, some soul-searching, and you will experience what a valuable resource a journal can be!

Healthy Habit for the Week

Each week, members are asked to focus on one specific healthy step that can be used on a daily basis. The step suggested in the workbook can be as simple as not eating on the run, or it can be an unbreakable commitment to drinking eight glasses of water a day. The idea is to make these steps a firm habit, a part of your daily life. Remember: if you focus on just one healthy habit each week, by the end of the program you will have ten healthy habits to help you keep going!

Reward for the Week

Rewarding yourself is a good way of acknowledging your success. Most people with a weight problem are very good at "beating themselves up" over it. An important part of creating the new you is to emphasize what you have achieved. The rewards suggested each week will help you do just that.

Team Activity for the Week

This section of your workbook gives you an imaginative suggestion every week that will help you and your teammates continue to bond. The suggestions are easy to do, fun, and will keep you on your toes!

Golden Rule for the Week

Sayings, proverbs, and rules are easy to remember, which is why every week you are asked to memorize a Golden Rule and make it your "mantra." These autosuggestions can have a huge impact on your behavior.

Foods of the Week

Each week you are given the complete profile of a healthy food to incorporate into your daily menus. You are told what it does for you in terms of your health; you are given recipe suggestions; and the food's nutritional value is explained. The range of healthy foods you eat regularly will greatly expand. By the end of the ten weeks, you will be munching on kale and steaming fish Chinese style!

Self-empowerment Exercise for the Week

Taking control of your eating will help you gain greater control over your life. The exercises in this section work on such crucial issues as self-image and self-esteem, which impact greatly your eating patterns.

Stress Antidote for the Week

When queried, Fight the Fat members listed stress as the No. 1 reason for overeating. This section offers a wide range of practical suggestions for dealing with stress without food. Not only will these exercises help you shed those extra pounds, but they will help create a calmer, healthier you!

A Great Deal for the Reader

If you can commit to ten weeks on the program, you will come out healthier and thinner, with new friends and closer ties to old ones. By the end of ten weeks, you will have started an exercise routine, tried new foods, and broken old self-destructive patterns. You will have chosen to live life to the fullest.

I came to Dyersville, Iowa, expecting to find a strictly local story. A New Yorker with a "tried everything, seen everything" attitude, I thought I'd get a few healthy recipes and maybe some exercise tips. What I discovered was the power of being there for another person and having another person be there for you. I came away inspired when I realized how much energy can be tapped when people get together and turn their lives around. Throughout the book, whenever I say, "I found out," or "I discovered," I am only passing on to you the cumulative wisdom and experience of Fight the Fat organizers Bobbi Schell, Dianna Kirkwood, and Jane Clemen. They became my "weight gurus" for a very simple reason: visiting Iowa, I saw for myself that Fight the Fat works.—Daniel Myerson

Chapter One: Town of Dreams

"A journey of a thousand miles begins with a single step...don't be overwhelmed by how far you have to go! Keep your eye on where you're coming from! Even if you haven't lost a pound—yet—you [got] off your couch and are sitting here at this meeting. Give yourself credit for this positive accomplishment!"
—Overheard at a Fight the Fat meeting.

On my first day in Dyersville, I went into the local McDonald's. After five minutes, I had to pinch myself to make sure I wasn't in a health spa. Nutrition tips were posted everywhere and Denise, the manager, was explaining the alternative menu, a feast of low-fat and healthy foods, to a customer. What's more, one of the employees was doing stretches as she waited for her next customer—she was part of an employee Fight the Fat team that was going up against Hardee's rival team, *The Starlites,* in this year's campaign.

The same thing was true of the Dyersville Subway. Brenda, the manager, was reeling off what seemed like an endless list of possibilities to a team of ten, the Dyersville *Bun Busters,* that had just come in together after exercising—each possibility she described sounded better than the next. The options were creative ways to vary the menu and maximize taste and minimize fat and calories (I'll get to them, and to the McDonald's menu, in the chapter on food, Week Seven).

Walking through town, I saw signs in food stores and restaurants, *We support Fight the Fat. Buy your low-fat foods here!* The LeRoy's Pizza had a *Low-fat Pizza* sign, and the Ritz Restaurant was offering a new healthy-for-your-heart, low-fat special—ostrich (raised locally). In Dyersville, if it is Tuesday it means ostrich (or bison, another healthy, low-fat meat making a come-back here. And the surprise is, it's really delicious!).

The *Millennium Grannies,* remarkably fit Dyersville matrons in their seventies and eighties (there are six of them), power walk past you (power walking requires you to pick up the pace and challenge yourself to increase your walking speed. See chapter five for details). If they stop it's not to catch their breath but to let a pair of bicyclers with *Love Handles* T-shirts whiz by (another Dyersville team composed of ten mothers).

In Dyersville everyone, and I am mean everyone, in town is into it—it being Fight the Fat. But why? How did it get started? And how can I, living in Brooklyn, join?

Those were some of the questions I posed to Bobbi Schell, Supervisor of Rehabilitation Outreach Services at Dyersville's Mercy Medical Center, after my stroll through town. Mercy is a not-for-profit Catholic hospital serving the tri-state area of Iowa, Wisconsin, and Illinois, particularly geared toward the rural areas. It was in one of those rural areas, Dyersville, where Fight the Fat originated. Mercy is known for its high-tech, state-of-the-art facilities, especially in regards to its rehabilitation and cardiac services, and its special commitment to the poor.

One of the original organizers, Bobbi, is a pretty brunette with a spring in her step and a bubbly laugh that makes everyone in a room smile the moment she enters it. When you first meet her, you are in for a shock: the first thought that goes through your mind is, "Look at her! You can be overweight *and* healthy!" This is from the energetic way she moves, from her stamina, and her great posture; it is obvious that she's healthy—everything about her reflects someone who is very much at home in her body.

That she is overweight is puzzling. But when you hear her talk, you realize that in another year or so, this woman definitely will not be carrying around any extra pounds. She is on the way, going from not being able to walk up a few steps carrying a bag of groceries to someone who gives exercise classes (shedding nearly fifty pounds in the process).

"Well—" she starts to answer my questions, but before she can get beyond the "well" she's interrupted by a telephone call. As she talks on the phone, she glances up at a bulletin board covered with slogans and suggestions and photos of her working out. The slogan she seems to be looking at reads *Give Your Troubles to God—He's Up All Night Anyway*. Obviously, the call is a difficult one—she's dealing with something about a budget crunch. And just as obviously, she's using the photos and the slogans on her bulletin board to help her. Later, I will discover that that is one of the Fight the Fat techniques—surround yourself with self-empowering slogans and images.

"No more calls, I promise!" she laughs, getting off the phone and taking a deep breath—she holds it for a good five seconds before resuming our interview (another Fight the Fat technique, I will learn later).

She explains, "Fight the Fat started as a way for people to get together with their friends or to make new friends who could help them in their struggle...Its mission was to tell people: you are not alone in your battle to get more healthy. It's not about being a size six or being able to run a marathon. It's about feeling good about yourself no matter what size you are. It is about being able to turn to people who can help you—and to help yourself by helping others. It's about not being too proud to take others' help. Being able to realize, I just can't do this on my own."

Realizing that teamwork was the key didn't happen overnight, Bobbi went on to explain—creating Fight the Fat was a step-by-step process. The first incentive was a Mercy survey that revealed that more than 50 percent of local health problems were weight related. So, Bobbi and her colleagues at Mercy, nutritionist Jane Clemen and Director of Marketing Dianna Kirkwood, put their heads together and got the community, the local radio station, the restaurants, and the recreation center involved. Before they knew it, from an avalanche of suggestions and good ideas, twenty-three teams were formed for the first Fight the Fat—they were on their way. "And it keeps evolving," Bobbi added with emphasis, "each year we discover ways to make it better."

More calls come in—questions about that day's schedule in Rehab and calls from her three school-age daughters.

"Do you mean to tell me," I ask with amazement, "that after a full day like this you give exercise classes at night?"

"This is the new me," she answers with a smile. "The truth is that ever since Fight the Fat began, I have so much more energy that when I look back at the old me it seems as if I was only half alive!"

This kind of energy surge is something you hear about again and again when talking to Fight the Fat participants. Nora is a thirty-six-year-old mother of five from nearby Balltown who invited me to join her on her power walk (she has been power walking for almost a year, ever since the first Fight the Fat). An enthusiastic woman who has taken off twenty-nine pounds and has thirty more to go, she alternates between maintaining and losing—and sometimes she even puts a few pounds back on.

"Progress is never a straight march forward," she tells me. "I learned not to get discouraged. Three steps forward, one step back, two forward is okay with me now. I mean, you meet some people who have lost a lot of weight at Fight the Fat and they all tell you that."

"What's the most valuable tip you've received from the others?" I ask. She answers right away, without hesitation: "Keep to your exercise regimen, no matter what slipups you have! Someone told me that during my first Fight the Fat and she was right. It's the way to go."

"What got you started?"

"To be honest, I joined because I wanted to look better. But now I feel so much better that there's no way I'd go back to my old habits. I knew I was putting on weight steadily although I refused to go on a scale, and this used to depress me. I wore clothes with elastic-band waists over blouses that I thought made me look thin. But I could feel how hard it was to do simple things like get out of a car. My son's high school graduation was coming up and I wanted him to be proud of me—that was one factor."

"And the others?" I asked, impressed by her ability to keep up a steady pace and talk at the same time—she was obviously in good shape.

"I help my husband out in business, he sells farm equipment, and he needed to do something about his weight as much as I did. I figured that if

I started it would influence him. So, I sat down and wrote him a letter telling him I wanted him to be alive to watch our kids grow up! He's not one to say much. He didn't answer me, but he took it in. When I told him I'd be going over to Dyersville for Fight the Fat with a carpool, he said no, he'd drive with me instead—he was coming to the meeting. It made me very happy."

"How has he benefited most?"

"Well, I think just listening to all the talk about good nutrition. My husband's the perfect example of a joke people tell around here. *You know you're an Iowan if you think of the four major food groups as beef, pork, beer, and Jell-O salad with marshmallows!* He hasn't joined officially, but he's picked up a lot secondhand, just the way some of the other husbands do. They sit home with their big beer bellies, and when the wives come back from the meetings they ask: 'What went on tonight?'"

In the beginning, Nora herself was slow to join Fight the Fat. Her sister Peg endlessly nagged at her, but that did no good until she saw that Peg had lost sixteen pounds. "That got me going all right," Nora remembers, going on to explain that her main excuse for not joining had been her family. She has children ranging in age from fourteen months to sixteen years. But Fight the Fat taught her that what is good for her ultimately will be good for them.

"They survive!" she laughs, describing the meals her teenagers cook on the nights she goes out to meetings. Plainly, they are not gourmet offerings—but just as plainly, the responsibility is good for her children who pull together as a family. While her children feast on scrambled eggs smothered in ketchup or tuna fish a la Sunkist, Nora makes a getaway to meet with her team, the *Meltaway Mommas.* They are a group composed of eight women who live either in Dyersville itself or in the nearby towns of Holy Cross and Balltown, and who vary greatly in ages and interests. But their commitment to Fight the Fat is strong enough to weld them together into one of the most successful teams.

"Now I won't give up my Fight the Fat nights for anything," Nora says as we walk together past a restaurant called Breitbach's, a place I'd heard about from many members. *The pies are so good here the governor has been known to send a state trooper two hundred miles for them.* But Nora barely gives it a glance.

Later, it is kickoff night of the third annual Fight the Fat—the meeting at which the basics of the program are explained. The members will hear the first of a series of talks by Mercy nutritionist Jane Clemen to help them plan that week's meals. Physical therapist Bobbi Schell will pass on some good advice about attitude and exercise. And organizer Dianna Kirkwood will introduce a Fight the Fat team that has prepared a skit to get things going on a fun note.

The Total Fitness Recreation Center on the south edge of Dyersville, soon to be filled with four hundred people, hums with activity. People pour into the hall from the town, from the surrounding countryside, and from nearby towns. Volunteers are putting last touches on decorations with weight-loss motifs: larger-than-life pictures of fruits and vegetables decorate one wall together with calorie counts underneath them, while a second wall is covered with life-size drawings of people exercising. Balloons and streamers and confetti hang from the ceiling, and posters with team logos hang over the various sections where the teams are to sit.

Fight the Fat has become a fact of life here in Dyersville, like the changing seasons or a national holiday. Everyone is psyched.

Peg, the team captain of the *Meltaway Mommas,* arrives and takes a seat in an empty row. "I have been waiting for tonight all year," she says, watching the door with anticipation for her teammates to arrive; she has designed the new team T-shirts and wants to see how they look in them. On the seat next to her is what she calls her "visual"—a ten-pound bag of lard.

"We all have to bring in something that weighs the amount we want to lose over the next ten weeks. And each week, as we take the pounds off our bodies, we bring in a lighter visual. By the last week, I hope I'll have gotten rid of every bit of *that,*" she points to the lard. "Some people bring in sugar, some bring in butter—it doesn't matter what as long as it helps you to actually see what you're carrying around."

Prompted to join because of back pain (her doctor said dropping twenty pounds would be the best medicine), she lost sixteen pounds during her first Fight the Fat and now has set ten more pounds as her goal. While in the past she had never been able to stay on a diet for more than a week or two, now the camaraderie has kept her going.

There is the sound of lively laughter as a team of eight friends comes into the room carrying a rope for the collective measurement of the team's waist. "I wasn't interested in joining in the beginning, although I had more than sixty pounds to lose," says Lotte, a cheerful brown-haired woman in her thirties with mischievous eyes. An aide at a nursing home, she had a new baby at home and a preschooler and worked a full eight-hour schedule—she felt that going to meetings at night would be too much for her. But, the example of a coworker at the nursing home changed her mind. Her colleague was a farm wife who came to work after getting up at four in the morning to milk the cows! "My attitude was," says Lotte, "if she can do it, so can I!"

Returning home from work exhausted, the only thing that got Lotte out to exercise was loyalty to her team, a Dyersville-based group of ten women called *Pounds Off.* "I'd force myself to go, feeling more dead than alive. But after working out forty minutes with my team—sometimes we'd even skip rope—I'd feel like a member of the human race again."

As Lotte talks, more people come in and the room echoes with the sound of excited exclamations. In one corner, a woman teaches a small group some new dance steps for a class they are taking together. In another, a team is doing some last minute practicing of their theme song.

At the back of the room, various tables have been set up where members can learn about things that may help them during the campaign. A massage therapist offers free five-minute massages for members who want to see if this relaxation method is for them. A woman from a store in nearby Dubuque gives out free samples of health foods for people to try. And the manager of a gym equipment store explains to interested members which of his products would be suitable for them.

Lotte's teammate Susan sits down beside her and gives her a hug. "They're going to be talking about the journal tonight," she says, waving to some more friends who are arriving. "It's not just a journal of what you ate during the day—it's kind of a diary that deals with overall questions. Its purpose is to help you get in touch with how you are feeling, and how you are doing. You can put anything you want in it. Are you ready to give up? Was work awful? Did your husband just leave? I mean, what's going on? People ask: what am I supposed to write in a journal? But there's no right or wrong. My journal will focus on what motivates me. You know, what lights my fire? When you know what that is, you will make it part of your life."

For those who hate to write, Fight the Fat organizer Jane Clemen has a neat suggestion. "Don't let that stop you! Get a small recorder (you can buy one cheap) and talk your thoughts into it. It doesn't matter how you do it, what matters is that you get out your feelings and your thoughts. It's good therapy."

Teammates start to take their seats together, and they call out friendly greetings and encouragement to rival teams. They all want to win, but they hope the other teams do well, too. The spirit of the competition is summed up by a large poster on the wall that reads *There is nothing noble in being superior to someone else. The true nobility is in being superior to your previous self.*

Large numbers of people keep arriving, singly, in couples, in threes and fours. There is noise, laughter, and the buzz of excited conversation as teammates and friends greet one another. Loud, rhythmic music begins. There is an explosion of applause and cheering. A voice announces over the loudspeaker: "Ladies and Gentlemen! Welcome to the third annual Fight the Fat!"

The battle has begun.

Your Workbook

The Bulletin Board

In a place where you can see it often (such as your kitchen or bedroom), put up a bulletin board where you can display helpful notices to yourself— it can be something as simple as a poster board. They can include inspirational thoughts that you read or heard at a Fight the Fat meeting, or they can be prayers that are meaningful to you, or simply jokes that cheer you up! If you glance at the bulletin board while you are making coffee in the morning or when you come home after a long day, you are giving yourself an extra dose of inspiration to help you through rough moments and tough choices.

"I have always insisted that slower is faster, whether you're trying to recover from an injury or start a ballet company. To succeed you must take deliberate steps with no shortcuts."
—Edward Villella, dancer and choreographer

"The tragedy is that so many people look for self-confidence and self-respect everywhere except within themselves, and so they fail in their search."
—Nathaniel Branden, psychologist

You might also want to post up on your bulletin board reminders of your overall goals as well as your goals, for the week and goals for the day. It might even be a very specific goal such as *Today I will park my car five blocks from work and walk the rest of the way,* or *Today I will have fruit instead of the cookies or candy passed around in the office.*

The bulletin board can also include healthy recipes you want to try. It can be a place where you want to pin before-and-after photos of yourself or friends.

You should also keep a Victory List here. The list will underline every step you take toward success. It might contain a notice like, *Went for a walk when I felt stressed out!* or, *Had a large salad and cottage cheese for lunch at work*…or, *No weight loss this week—but made healthier choices in what I ate.*

We tend to overlook our successes and harp on our failures. Becoming aware that we are taking small but important steps towards our goals reinforces our new behavior. Just as small amounts of money eventually add up to large ones, so small victories add up to a new healthier you. As the weeks go on, the list will get longer, and just reading it over and/or sharing it with a teammate will help improve the way you see yourself. By setting up your Bulletin Board right away, at the beginning of week one, you are setting yourself up for victory.

More Food...for Thought

"Who are mighty? They who conquer themselves."
—Hebrew saying from *Ethics of the Fathers*

"All beginnings are hard."
—Spanish proverb

"All virtue is habit."
—Marcus Aurelius

"Habit is either the best of servants or the worst of masters!"
— Nathaniel Emmos

This quote came courtesy of a grandma who in the 1930s taught in an Iowa one-room rural schoolhouse. She offered this gem before heading out to umpire at her granddaughter's softball game:

"Though you may have difficulty exercising in the beginning,
remember—repetition is the mother of skill!"
—Sue Engelbrecht, RN at Mercy Medical Center

A Reminder

At the turn of the millennium, there were a lot of lists. Einstein was the man of the century. Ruth and Jordan were the athletes of the century, and so on. Well they missed one. How about the millennium's most significant organ? The heart beats a couple of billion times in a lifetime. Even at rest, the heart can circulate the entire body's blood supply in one minute. In an athlete, it can do this up to six times a minute. This amazing pump replaces itself, molecule by molecule, once every six months. Think of that. You have in your chest the organ of the millennium! Take good care of it!

If You Need to Be Scared

The Metropolitan Life Insurance Company put these statistics out to spread the word:

Death Rate Goes Up With Each Excess Pound

Among moderately overweight men, the death rate is
42 percent higher than among men of normal weight.

Among very overweight men, the death rate is
81 percent higher than among men of normal weight.

Among moderately overweight women, the death rate is
42 percent higher than among women of normal weight.

Among very overweight women, the death rate is
61 percent higher than among women of normal weight.

Your Journal

(Remember: you can *talk* your answers into a recording machine or write them out, whichever way is more comfortable for you.)

The following focus question can help you start off your journal for week one—but don't limit yourself to this suggested topic. Use your journal as your personal sounding board. It's your psychiatrist, your best friend, your rabbi or priest—and your accountant and lawyer!—all rolled into one. It will help you let off steam, understand yourself better, and keep a record of your progress. When you're down in the dumps, just reviewing your earlier struggles will make it easier to go on.

When you're feeling good and want to record some victory or triumph that would otherwise have been forgotten (*I passed up the cheesecake! I've really gotten into weight lifting! I'm beginning to like my new way of eating more than the old!*) this is the place to write it down. Over time, your journal can become a powerful new force in your life. It will be your friend, the encouraging voice that tells you *Look at what you can do!*

With that said, consider this question: *Why is it that I am not making healthy choices?* Compare situations where you have opted for health with those where you have let yourself go to the dogs.

Give yourself time to think about the question, writing whatever comes to mind on the page. If nothing comes to mind, keep writing, until your associations begin to flow. Just the activity of sitting and writing will trigger thoughts.

The journal is one way that you can begin to get to know yourself. It's a simple technique, but a powerful one. Make use of it and compare notes with your teammates (skip any sections that you want to keep private). You will see in a short time how much you had to learn—about yourself!

Healthy Habit for the Week

Hey! I'm not hungry! I'm thirsty!
No! More than thirsty—I'm dehydrated!
It's all right to drink like a fish—if you drink what a fish drinks!

Eight glasses of water daily (64 ounces). The water can be hot or cold, or spiked with lemon or lime. It can be in the form of decaffeinated teas or non-caloric seltzer, which comes in a wide variety of delicious natural flavors (Note: beverages containing caffeine cannot be counted as part of the daily total.)

There are literally hundreds of herbal teas out there with flavors that range from spicy ginger to soothing chamomile. Let the tea bags steep for a long while to get a stronger flavor; when the water cools slightly, the tea is at its best. You are satisfying your taste buds and helping your body accomplish what it needs to get done. Water will help promote the burning of fat, help cleanse the system during weight loss, is itself a diuretic, and will help eliminate bloating due to water retention.

A glass of water before a meal can take the edge off your hunger. And perhaps most important: the more water the better as a means of helping prevent bladder cancer. Six eight-ounce glasses of water a day reduces the risk of bladder cancer by 50 percent, according to a study by Dr. Dominique Michaud at the Harvard School of Public (New England Journal of Medicine, May 6th, 1999).

Reward for the Week

No more oversize shirts and stretch pants! You care about how you look! So *now* turn these words into action. Focus on your body—buy yourself something you know makes you look hot. Whatever it is—clothing, jewelry, a hat, a scarf—choose it with care. You're saying: *the way I look matters to me. I am important to myself.* Arrange to do this with a team member or two (how many times do we put off—forever—something we mean to get to?). This way, you're locked into a date and a time. Plus, it will be more fun to go together. There are hundreds of ways you can bond with your team members. This is a great one.

Team Activity for the Week

Sharing Inspiration. Let everyone on your team bring in an inspiring story—*at least* one, the more, the better. It doesn't have to be about weight loss. It can focus on the life of a famous person whose belief in their inner strength was vindicated. Or it can be about a relative, a neighbor, or someone you know who would not give up. What qualities made for their success? How can that be applied to your own life, especially to your participation in Fight the Fat? Or, you may want to have your story focus on examples of what has been achieved through team spirit and community action.

You'll find that preparing to talk about such a story to your teammates will make you dwell on the details, on the step-by-step process of success. The lessons you learn, and teach, will have a greater impact on you than if you merely read through them in a book. This kind of teamwork is a great way of making real-life lessons hit home and impact your day-to-day decisions.

Golden Rule for the Week

Watch out for fat as well as calories! And watch out for calories as well as fat! You can reduce fat by being vigilant! Just take the following simple steps and you will reduce your fat intake by more than half:

- Bake or broil meats instead of frying them.
- Double-rinse ground beef and blot patties.
- Pull the skin off chicken and trim fat off meats.
- Use butter and margarine sparingly. Measure these ingredients out as if you were on a deserted island and they were part of your last supplies.
- Use low-fat salad dressings and measure out the amount you use with spoons—don't just pour it on.
- Limit the amount of meat you eat. Three ounces of meat twice a day is the max. Try other excellent sources of protein, such as fish, tofu, rice, and beans (there are many great recipes for these!).

- Know about the foods you are eating. Get the fat content as well as the calorie count. *Low-calorie does not automatically mean low-fat. And low-fat does not automatically mean low-calorie!*

Food of the Week

Get used to adding barley to your menu. Barley? Why?
Ever see the movie *Gladiator?*

If you have, I don't have to tell you about those big brawny guys fighting to the death. What did they eat? Well, in ancient times they were called *hordearii*—barley eaters!

That was the secret of their strength! Barley provides all the complex carbohydrates you need without giving you the fat you get in meat. It also gets points as a source of fiber and protein. Studies have shown that eating barley lowers cholesterol by up to 15 percent and promotes weight loss!

You can use barley instead of rice in many recipes. Or, you can mix it with rice or cook it in soups. Mushroom and barley soup, for example, is delicious *and* really healthy. I smelled the following version of it cooking as I walked down the street in Brooklyn and it smelled so good I thought I would faint. I had the audacity to knock on the door and ask for the recipe. Here it is from the kitchen of Mrs. Belle P.—a tried and true soup that will get you ready for your next appearance in the gladiator ring. It's as simple as it is delicious:

Mushroom and Barley Soup a la Brooklyn
1 large onion
½ cup barley
½ cup lentils (optional)
1 10-ounce container of mushrooms
3 carrots

3 stalks of celery
2 cloves of garlic
One parsnip
Parsley and Dill (to taste)
Salt and Pepper (to taste)
6–7 cups of water

1) Dice the onion, carrots, celery, and parsnip. Sauté the onion and the garlic in a teaspoon of olive oil until soft.
2) Add water, barley, lentils, sautéed onion and garlic, and diced vegetables.
3) Cook over a small flame until the lentils and barley are soft (an hour or more).
4) Enjoy!
Note: Quick-cooking barley (10 minutes)
  (Regular pearled barley takes 40 minutes)

Here's another barley-rich recipe that might tickle your taste buds. This recipe was found in *Vegetarian Times,* February 2001, and has received high grades in the taste department from Fight the Fat organizer Dianna Kirkwood. She adds this word of advice, "Pearled barley should be stored in an airtight container, and whole barley in addition needs to be kept in the fridge to play it safe!"

Southwestern Barley
1 10-ounce package of frozen baby lima beans
One cup quick-cooking barley
One medium red bell pepper, thinly sliced
⅓ cup tomato juice
3 tbsp. fresh lime juice
2 tbsp. olive oil
2 tbsp. chopped cilantro

One clove garlic, minced
One tsp ground cumin
One tsp dried oregano
½ tsp hot pepper sauce

1) Cook lima beans according to package directions; drain and cool.
2) In medium saucepan, bring 3 cups water to a boil.
3) Add barley and cook until tender, 10 minutes. Drain, rinse under cold water, and drain again, pressing to remove excess moisture.
4) Transfer barley to medium bowl. Add lima beans and red pepper.

In a small bowl, mix it up! Tomato juice, lime juice, oil, cilantro, garlic, cumin, oregano, and hot sauce. Add salt to taste. Pour dressing over barley mixture and toss to blend. Serve at room temperature.

(252 calories, 7 grams fat)

Self-empowerment Exercise for the Week

Drawing on past achievements. We all have accomplished things in life that we take for granted. But these achievements required self-discipline, self-control, staying power, and skill. For example, studying for and passing a school exam; learning how to play a musical instrument; learning how to quilt; and learning how to speak a foreign language. Some of us have given up smoking. Some haven't missed a single week in synagogue or church for months. If you've spent a night nursing an ailing parent or child or spouse, if you've gotten up every morning at four A.M. to milk a cow or at six A.M. to commute to work, you have "it," willpower that you can now tap for your *new* goal—you.

We have done things as difficult as weight loss—so we should face this challenge with more confidence if we make a list of our "forgotten" accomplishments and take a moment to realize how much we are capable of *when we want to be!* Share this list with teammates. A session devoted to confidence boosting can be just what you need to get you through your next exercise session. It is your sense of who you are that permits you to achieve success.

Stress Antidote for the Week

Too often, our answer to stress is to put something in our mouths—it's simple, it's fast, we don't have to think, we don't have to deal with things. But there are other non-food ways of combating stress that leave us in control of the situation. Turning to non-food ways of nourishing ourselves doesn't leave us with a sugar "hangover" the next day and that "Oh my God! What have I done to myself?" feeling when we face the mirror. The key is to develop deeply satisfying *non-food* activities that inspire, enliven, and replace the cure-all that sugar and fast foods have become. If you get in the habit of incorporating even just one of the antistress techniques from this book into your life, you have taken a giant step forward towards creating the new, healthier, slimmer you.

The first antistress technique given below seems so simple, so basic, and so far away from the world of gyms and health foods that you might ask yourself, "What does this have to do with anything?" But try it and you will see! Remember, for the overweight, eating is in the head, not the stomach! Eating has ceased to have much to do with the body (when was the last time you ate because you were really hungry or faint from lack of food?). That's why many of the suggestions are for your brain—not your stomach! Okay, with that in mind, here it goes:

Take a few moments to write down ten blessings in life, large and small, that we take for granted. Share what you've written with your teammates. Each member is sure to come up with an awesome list that will complement yours. The energy from this kind of a session lasts a lot longer than a sugar rush, and permanently changes the way you look at things as well. This exercise allows you to take the focus off where you want to be, what you want to do, and what you want to have in life, and puts it on what has already been given to you.

P.S.: Keep in mind when you read the stress-reduction suggestions during the following weeks that whatever method you choose, it will require *time!* It takes time to calm down, and it takes time to shift the focus. It means pausing in the midst of frantic activity and rushed days.

Take the advice of Fight the Fat member Dianna Kirkwood, a busy executive with four children and numerous responsibilities. "Make time for yourself! That is what I have learned. No more skipping lunch, no more working without breaks! I have learned to walk away from the office with a half-dozen unanswered messages and a pile of papers cluttering my desk. I might spend an hour chatting with a friend or relaxing with a great book. In the long run, it makes me a more efficient worker and a more in-control person. It has helped me stop eating due to being mentally exhausted.

"My motto is," she adds, *"No one is going to die over this!* Actually, if I didn't have that motto, I might be the one dying!"

Chapter Two: Your Own Dyersville

Never underestimate the power of a group!
—Fight the Fat slogan

You can create a Fight the Fat campaign of your own provided you understand the goal. Forget about being rigid, and forget copying every part of the program. At the end of the day, it doesn't matter how you do it, how many people are involved, and what your activities are. What matters is that you get the spirit of Dyersville's Fight the Fat. That's the magic ingredient.

What you need is a little imagination and the desire to change your life. Your will to change, to make use of all of your potential, is immediately multiplied by 100 percent the minute you team up with even one other person. That connection, that vital link, gives your quest an added boost. Now you are doing it for another person as well as yourself, and that makes all the difference. You may seem crazy to your friends and family, but you are not crazy to your teammate—and the two of you together can face anything down.

Teammates

So, who are you going to recruit for your team? You may want to work with just one other empathic person you know and like and have much in common with. But working with people that you do not know well or only know in one situation also has its benefits. As Fight the Fat member Laura of Monticello, Iowa, said, "You think you know someone, but you really don't. There were women I had talked to at work, in church, and in a carpool…to take the kids to day camp. But then you begin getting to know them as teammates and it's just amazing…the kinds of things that come up. We began by talking about light stuff—you know, recipes and how hard it is to exercise. But after a while we felt more secure with each other. We trusted each other. When you are fighting together with a problem that's been dragging you down for a long time, you feel for your teammate. When she has a success, you begin to feel as if it's yours. I never thought it would work that way, but it does."

She continued, "I won't talk to my husband anymore about my weight—I know the kind of reaction I'll get. He's heard about it for years from me and doesn't really want to hear it anymore even though he listens. But I'll call up my teammate because she is struggling, too. She knows where I'm at. She cares in a different way."

If you decide to open up your team to whomever wants to join, remember that weight is an issue for everyone from teenagers to seniors, from rich to poor, from the high-pressured executive mom to the stay-at-home parent. Once you start the ball rolling, you become a magnet attracting countless others. Since word-of-mouth will bring many friends-of-friends into the picture, you must decide in advance exactly how large a group you are prepared to include. This year, the organizers of the Dyersville Fight the Fat set a cutoff number (and a cutoff date to register). So, nearby towns have started their own programs for those who were left out.

In Iowa, it wasn't only Dyersville, but five neighboring towns that became the community for Fight the Fat. People here had a lot in common—many were farmers or came from farming backgrounds and had gone to school together. The shared values that made it natural to tackle the weight problem as a town.

But let's expand our idea of a "team" to include you and one other person. Let's stretch our idea of community to include the people you meet at the Laundromat. Suddenly you will "know" all sorts of people—people who you don't *really* know and who could easily start up a team with you.

Take two couples who meet for the movies and eating out every week. If they are huffing and puffing when they get up from the table, all it takes is one forward-looking person to say, *Look, let's keep the movie part of our friendship, but change the heavy meal afterwards to a brisk walk and a light meal.* That represents the start of teamwork, of bonding for a positive goal. You can add other elements (and maybe other members) as you go along.

Or, they can be parents of children who go to the same school as your children. Private schools frequently organize fund-raisers; why not make that the occasion to sound out the other parents about Fight the Fat? In this way, you can do something for yourself at the same time that you are helping your children. If you are a senior, your focus group can be the other members of your senior citizen center.

People from different backgrounds can also bond. It's a question of striking a good balance. One of the teams in the Iowa Fight the Fat is made up of women of all ages and at different stages in their lives, from young mothers to empty nesters. The sharing of different perspectives is one of the strengths of the group. A factor making things easier for them, though, was geography: they all lived within ten minutes of each other. Meetings could be frequent and were easy to attend.

If you live in a large city, you might want to think about geography, too. The people that live in a ten- or twenty-block radius or even just in your apartment building can be a good starting point.

That's what my friend Fran tried, asking me to join her (for moral support) on the night she decided to canvass her neighbors in Sheepshead Bay, Brooklyn. She knocked on doors in her apartment building and introduced herself as peepholes clicked open. The responses ranged from a gruff, "What do you want?" to "No one's at home!" (we got *three* of those) to "Could you come back some other time—I'm eating!"

We switched our strategy and put up notices. To our surprise, on the night we had announced a meeting to explore the possibilities, sixteen people showed up. Fran was prepared with some "deals" she had been offered. The owner of a local fish store offered to grill any fish a member bought for no extra charge (strictly an eat-out proposition, though, since she had no restaurant license). The manager of a nearby YMCA offered to let the group use a room for meetings on a weekly basis; he was also receptive to discussing group benefits if they decided to join. And the local florist promised to donate a thirty-dollar bouquet of flowers as a prize for the member who lost the most weight. There it was, *a beginning*.

So far, Fran has kept her group small—it is just Fran and four other members. They meet at each other's apartments, which makes it very convenient. And during the spring, they plan to go up to the roof together to do stretches and some mild ("very mild" she says with emphasis) exercise.

"We haven't taken the florist up on his offer," says Fran, "because we're not sure we want to do the competition thing—yet. Maybe we'll never get around to it. But we do weigh in at the meetings. And fish consumption in this apartment building is definitely on the rise as opposed to fatty meats."

By the time you read this, *Fran & Co.* will have added more elements because that's just the way Fight the Fat works: the enthusiasm builds. It gathers momentum like a rock rolling down a hill.

A weekly Fight the Fat newsletter for your group is another great idea—with the computer, it is easy to send out emails or to print out twenty or thirty copies of a "How Are We Doing?" or a "Fat Fighters Manifesto" where you list your goals and highlight the achievements of group members. The point is that getting together a Fight the Fat campaign does not have to be overwhelming.

When relaxing in a chat room on the Internet, suggest to a cyberspace friend that you swap health suggestions, or keep a weight chart together! Again, starting a program does not mean putting every piece of the puzzle together right away.

That's how the Dyersville Fight the Fat started: a few simple measures taken by three women who were concerned about their health and the health of their friends and family. They had no idea that before they were through, they would be attracting national attention!

The organizers of Fight the Fat in Dyersville were busy women who all held full-time jobs and who had husbands, children, and, in two cases, elderly parents demanding their attention. They could commit just so much time, and no more to Fight the Fat, but they found that the project had instant appeal—it touched a nerve in many people.

Bobbi, one of the guiding spirits of the program who was enthusiastic from the word go, said, "You make a few calls or send a few emails and before you know it, so many people are involved!"

"How did you know who to call at first?" I asked, wanting to understand what was behind her success.

"I didn't," she shrugged. "I tried everyone I could think of. I asked people for suggestions. Sometimes I would explain what I was trying to do to whomever picked up the phone...they told me who to call in their organization.

"You'd be surprised at how many people feel desperate about their weight. But they don't do anything about it because it's too hard for them to get started on their own. Once I had a core of people at the medical center that felt the same way I did, I knew we would succeed. It's like throwing a pebble into a pool of quiet water—the ripple effect is very powerful."

"Give me an example," I asked her. "How did you approach the very first person you called?"

"Well, that was Jane. I said to her, 'You know, Jane, there are things that I know I will do for my friends and my family that I just won't do for myself. So, if you and I got together and agreed to support each other in switching to a healthy lifestyle, I know it will help keep me going. I would be watching myself, watching my diet, my exercise...not just for myself, but for you, too.' That made sense to her and she agreed to join me in figuring out a program. Since then, the "doing-it-together" principle has proven true for a lot of other people as well. It is like a team bonding together in sports— the team members achieve more than they normally would have because they cheer each other on. You make it through the week because you want to be able to step off the scale and tell your friends, 'I've lost this week!' You know how good you will feel. You just don't want to let them down."

"I'm a very private person," says Jane Clemen, the very dedicated and knowledgeable nutritionist at Mercy who helped Bobbi set the town on fire. "But I like a challenge. I like dealing with people and trying something new. Making those first calls turned out to be fun. I would sound out the people with a few simple questions I drew up in advance. Basically, my first concern was to talk to people that I knew could help sponsor the event. 'Would you be interested in joining a community effort to achieve health and fitness?' I would ask after introducing myself. And almost all of the people I called were very positive."

June, one of the organizing committee members, talked about one of her experiences, "When I first called the Chamber of Commerce to get them involved in Fight the Fat, a lady there (who had failed on scores of diets, I found out later) asked me in exasperation, 'What difference do you think teaming up will make?' And I told her, 'Today I'm going to the recreation center for my first aerobics class. Alone it would be hard for me to go to a gym looking the way I look—I'm more than fifty pounds overweight. But I know that my other teammates will be just as out of shape as I am! I know that the instructor will be gearing the class to people like me. I'll be in an environment that's friendly and supportive. I won't be looking to the right and left and seeing slim women in leotards stretching their legs over their heads. I'll be seeing teammates who are determined to make a new start. That's why! Any questions?' There was a pause—and then she asked me, 'How can I join?'"

Another important lesson Fight the Fat organizers learned is that groups receive special consideration that individuals don't. Even a single team of seven or eight people who regularly eat at a restaurant will be able to work out helpful arrangements. If the manager of a pizza parlor or restaurant knows that team members will be coming in regularly after exercise sessions, he will be sure to accommodate the needs of the team. He will have the kind of pizza requested, made with low-fat mozzarella and a thin crust; or he will work out an alternative Fight the Fat menu (often one that lists fat grams and calorie counts as well as prices!). And he might even come up with an interesting meal of his own.

One restaurateur I talked to in Iowa had come up with a vegetarian platter that was just delicious. She used all kinds of spices and sauces and created a dish she called Vegetable Heaven that was better than some of the high-calorie meals on her menu. Proof: customers who didn't have to lose weight ordered it. "After all, these people are making money by providing for us," organizer Dianna Kirkwood exclaimed. "Why shouldn't they give us what we need?"

I liked Dianna's theory so much that I thought I would ask a friend of mine, Lisa, to try it out in the Manhattan office where she worked (the high-pressure office of a major advertising firm where crises are the order of the day). Regularly at 10 A.M., a young man appeared there wheeling in a little cart with coffee and snacks: danishes, doughnuts, muffins—empty calories with little nutritional value and lots of sugar that would provide a temporary rush and then leave everyone feeling bummed out. I asked Lisa to see whether she could get fellow workers interested in having other things on that cart like fruits and juices, *low-fat* muffins, health bars, and other low-calorie or healthy snacks.

"Once I'd brought up the subject, I was really surprised," Lisa reported back a week later. "Not only were the nine overweight people in the office gung ho for the idea, but I learned that even people who you would never imagine had a weight problem struggled *so hard* to keep from 'bloating up' as they put it. They might only have ten or fifteen pounds to shed, but they knew that ten or fifteen pounds have a way of turning into twenty or thirty before you know it (that would make a good advertising slogan, wouldn't it?).

"The boss liked the idea, too, although, as a rule, let me tell you he's a little Napoleon and very negative about anyone telling him what to do in the office. So, when he's for something, that's a victory. I guess everybody is more health conscious these days. Why not have foods with nutritional value on the cart? Nobody was against it—even those who dearly loved their sugar doughnuts said that they were willing to try something new."

Location

For those groups that are committed from the beginning to exercising together, joining a recreation center provides a great solution. It's often a perfect place to meet before or after exercising. Mary Wessels, the director of the recreation center in Dyersville, felt that Fight the Fat was one of the best things that had happened in Dyersville. She did everything she could to support the program from the start. "Many new members forty years and older have joined. We have a dancercize class now and older-on-up classes. We make sure that the orientations are one on one so that people won't feel intimidated and so that we can talk about their particular concerns. We place them in the class that's just right for them—it's hard to be the only overweight or older person in a group."

She added, "And there's the camaraderie that teams provide—I've seen the difference when really out of shape or overweight people join by themselves and when they join as a team. Believe me, the team members are much better at sticking to it over a long period of time. They joke around and keep each other going when things get hard. Plus, we have discounts for groups—really good deals that people can decide on after they've had a few classes and feel comfortable."

You can also decide to use libraries and bookstores for meeting places. Large chain stores like Barnes and Nobles and Borders often schedule author readings and have excellent spaces where meetings can take place. Books from their motivational, weight loss, nutrition, and health and fitness sections can be used as focal points of these discussions. Everyone benefits (including the store from sales), and you have a great location. The same thing is true of libraries. I asked an upstate New York librarian if she would let a group have a meeting room in the library for this purpose, and she agreed with the condition that they would become "friends of the library" (at $5 per year per member, that was a bargain).

Whether you schedule your meetings in a bowling alley or piggyback them on your PTA meetings ("Will all Fight the Fat members please remain!"), the goal is to jump start your Fight the Fat campaign; don't wait for the ideal spot. Just get this first crucial step in place. Later on, as the membership grows, you may choose to change the meeting place. The main thing is to get started.

Sources of Information

Another important decision you must make early on is what your sources of information will be. How will you learn about nutrition and exercise? How will you keep motivated as a group?

In Dyersville, Mercy Medical Center provided the expertise. This book is a good start, and in addition a list of helpful books is provided at the end (along with speakers you can invite to address your meeting, if your group is large enough). Your group may decide to watch an inspirational video together or they may opt to attend an announced lecture about stress reduction given in a local university or meditation center—one of those events that you never quite got to on your own.

Important: whatever your sources of information, make sure that you and your group refer to works written by acknowledged professionals in the health field. Many times, overweight people have the willpower, but don't have the patience to learn the calorie values and the fat content of the foods they eat. Or they misunderstand the relationship between exercise and weight loss.

One woman assumed that because she was eating healthy snacks—yogurt covered raisins, dried fruit, and nuts—she couldn't go wrong (she ended up gaining two and a half pounds on the first week of her "diet"). Another man assumed that because he was walking twenty minutes every night, he didn't have to worry so much about what he was eating. This kind of misconception was quickly put to rest by a speaker who quoted the book *Walking Off Weight. You have to walk the entire length of a football field to work off one M&M!*

Expenses

Finally, covering expenses is a factor that should not be left out of the equation: *it is important to charge all the participants a membership fee.* Not only does the money prove to be useful in terms of financing creative events, it also has a psychological effect. People value what they pay for. They tend to discount what comes free. The member who has spent thirty dollars to join Fight the Fat will be less likely to skip the meeting, and will be more committed to the effort. You might have a basic membership fee and then organize special events, like a night out dancing or a weekend walking tour for which there is a separate charge.

In downtown Los Angeles, for example, the historical society sponsors an amazing walking tour that includes the palatial movie theaters from the 1920s, marble and gilt extravaganzas that are usually kept closed to the public. New York City also has a walking tour sponsored by the city's historical society—you burn up calories while following the docent from sight to sight, meet interesting people, learn about the city's history—a fun way to exercise and a group activity that helps the team bond together for a very low fee.

This kind of active, non-food weekend event helps get the team members through those first weekends, which can be the most difficult times. Free time can spell trouble since new habits have not yet been formed and the old eat-your-way-through-the-weekend syndrome has not yet been changed to bicycle-your-way from Friday afternoon to Sunday!

Important Steps

In putting together your Fight the Fat campaign, you may want to begin by interviewing community leaders, recreation center managers, hospital directors, and health care givers in your community.

Perhaps the most important step in creating your own Fight the Fat is to explain to a potential member the unique value of the team spirit and the team meetings. If overweight and out-of-shape people could have seen what I did during my visit to Iowa, they would understand what a wonderful solution exists for their problem. There is simply no describing the energy-charged meetings in which you can see the determination and enthusiasm on the faces of the participants. There is electricity in the air.

During one of these Fight the Fat meetings in Dyersville, a remarkably fit woman named Peg made room for me to sit down next to her. "Look around you," she whispered to me. "These meetings do something to you. It's not just what you learn at them, although you do learn a lot. It's not just the fun we have, although that's something I look forward to. But you really feel as if you get a big shot of *willpower* during the meeting that keeps you going for the whole week. People can give you all kinds of good advice in your life, and you hear them, you know, but you don't *really* hear them. You don't take it in. At the meetings, the atmosphere kind of opens you up and makes you *really* listen. You realize that you are fighting for your life."

"If you could pass on one piece of advice or tip that has helped you the most," I asked her, "what would it be?"

"A speaker said during my first Fight the Fat meeting last year, *We can either let our appetites control us or we can control our appetites*. What she said, but even more important, the way that she said it, and the way that everyone cheered afterwards, made a big impression on me. I will never forget it. That was thirty-two and a half pounds ago."

Your Workbook

Exercises, Questions, Tips, & Points to Ponder for Week 2 of Fight the Fat

The Bulletin Board

"Problems don't have to make you binge on food.
But bingeing always causes problems!"
—Kay Sheppard, author of *Food Addiction*

"Modern medicine is a wonderful thing, but there are two problems.
People expect too much of it and too little of themselves."
—Don Ardell

More Food...for Thought

Why not think about your health when you still have it? Some of the steps suggested in this book, such as trimming away the fat from meats, drinking eight glasses of water per day, and taking that morning walk or that lunchtime run, do not require superhuman willpower or effort. They are very simple habits that quickly become second nature and make all the difference.

"Finish each day and be done with it. You have done what you could;
some blunders and absurdities have crept in; forget them as soon as you can.
Tomorrow is a new day; you shall begin it serenely and with too high a
spirit to be encumbered with your old nonsense."
— Ralph Waldo Emerson

"Change your thoughts, and you change your world."
—Norman Vincent Peale

"If not now, when?"
—Hebrew saying

There is never a perfect time to begin to diet and exercise. There will always be a reason to put it off. Make that reason—whatever it is—a good time to start.

Your Journal

**"I have always wanted to be somebody,
but I see now I should have been more specific!"**
—Lily Tomlin

Keep the following questions in mind during the entire week. *Let the answers suggest themselves to you:*

1) *What is my goal?*
2) *What concrete steps do I need to take to achieve it?*
3) *How will I feel when I succeed?*
4) *How will I change for the better when I succeed?*

Setting specific, reachable goals is a key to success. Once you achieve these, you can go on to the next level, and then the next, in your goal setting.

Meeting that first reasonable challenge, and achieving that first goal, is really empowering. When you are clear on exactly where you want to go and how you will get there and in what period of time you will manage this, you are already a different person from the old you.

It doesn't matter whether you have twenty or sixty pounds to lose—the moment you say, "In two weeks time I will have walked three times a week for thirty minutes a session," you are no longer drifting. You have broken up that huge unmanageable goal into a clearly defined hurdle and you can take on that challenge and win!

Get the momentum going! Set a goal!

Compare notes with your teammates. Don't forget: another person struggling with the same problem will provide strength just by being there for you. And you will get strength by being there for them. Also keep in mind that *your goals can change constantly throughout Fight the Fat*. If becoming more active is an early goal, the level or type of activity can gradually increase. Change of lifestyle goals is the all-time winner—pounds go and pounds come, but a healthier lifestyle is forever!

It is a good idea to carry the above questions and answers with you and read them over when you feel discouraged or tempted. By reading them you will hear your own voice when you were in an upbeat and sane mood—it might be just what prevents a binge!

Healthy Habit for the Week

Cut back on salt. Salt retains up to seventy times its weight in water, and excess fluids can make you look puffy. Australian researchers say that the number and size of the holes in your saltshakers can make a big difference since people "apply a similar manual action to all shakers"—that is, they shake just as hard whether the holes are small or large! Now who would have thought of that?

Some like it hot! Use pepper and spices instead to give your food that added flavor. Spicy food slows you down: you simply can't wolf down highly seasoned food the way you can wolf down bland dishes. And, by slowing down your pace, you tend to eat less. As an example, look at the small highly spiced dishes offered in many Indian restaurants. A few spoonfuls of each dish leaves you satisfied.

Keeping the health factor in mind will help motivate you. Salt causes you to retain water (giving you that bloated look) and has also been linked to hypertension and high blood pressure. High blood pressure is one of the "silent killers." As a Mercy Medical Center nurse reminds us: "I was in a drug store the other day and noticed one of those automatic blood pressure machines. You sit down, slide in your arm, push a button, and have your blood pressure in about one minute. As I get older, knowing my blood pressure keeps getting easier and easier, as the importance gets more and more crucial. Check it out."

Reward for the Week

You're going to be surprised by this one! It doesn't sound like a reward, but believe me, it'll end up giving you more pleasure and satisfaction than you can imagine.

Outward Directed Energy—A Great Solution for Weight Loss

Plan one team meeting that will be devoted to helping the less fortunate in your community. By throwing yourself into an activity that will help others, you will take your mind off your weight and shed those pounds faster. Are there kids who need someone to take them on an outing? What about reading for the blind? Visiting the sick in your local hospital or the elderly in a nursing home? Taking time out of our busy schedule to help someone is actually a great way to regain a sense of perspective: we are thankful that our problems are no worse than they are. In addition, such activities are very satisfying. We return to our own lives renewed and refreshed.

Doctor Tedd Mitchell, director of the Cooper Clinic's Wellness Program in Dallas, outlines the emotional as well as physical boost we get from helping others in an article for *HealthSmart* and concludes by observing, "We were not made to live solitary lives. Unfortunately, too many of us think of ourselves first. The irony is that by emphasizing our own needs instead of caring for others, we hurt ourselves in the long run."

Team Activity for the Week

"I could have danced all night!"
—*My Fair Lady*

"Dance is the poetry of the foot."
—John Dryden

A great advantage of team membership is that it makes it easier to try new activities.

If you are scared of feeling out of place or of looking silly in a dance class, the team support is a terrific way to overcome these negative feelings. If you can't get the whole team to go along with you on this one, then one or two teammates will do just as well. Including dance in your life can be what the doctor ordered. On a gray day when you are feeling down, what is more fun than trying out new steps, letting your body move to the rhythm of music, forgetting *everything* but the present moment?

Sound enticing? Especially if it's something the old you would not have considered trying in a million years, you should give it a whirl. The point of Fight the Fat is to break old mind-sets. Start a new pattern! You can opt for beginner's classes in ballroom dancing, jazz, modern dance, belly dancing (what fun!), even ballet or flamenco. One member recommended seeing the movie *Strictly Ballroom* to get you going. "I took it out on video and found it inspiring. All those people obsessed with music and movement—they make you want to start dancing right there as you're watching them."

Find the class that's right for you and you'll be learning about a new art form, listening to music, getting in touch with your body, and, incidentally, burning up calories! Classes usually start with warm-ups and stretches that relax the mind and body. And then the fun begins!

To find out which classes are offered near you, call local dance studios or check with the Continuing Education Department of your local colleges. An eight-week course can cost as little as sixty dollars and the results, both in terms of your morale and your waist line, are worth every penny.

Joyce, an early Fight the Fat member, joined a line dancing group and reports that they have gotten so good they perform throughout the state. "I'm trying to shift my attention from my stomach to my feet!" she jokes, adding that when her group performs at a nursing home or hospital it is one of the highlights of her year.

Golden Rule for the Week

Never eat on the run! Don't even eat standing! Sit down and enjoy what you eat—it will make every bite last longer!

Don't watch TV, read the newspaper, or talk on the telephone while you eat. Savor every bite! And chew, chew, chew, chew! Madelaine, of Balltown, Iowa, says: "I don't allow any upsetting discussions or fights at the dinner table. If the phone rings, I will never take it. For me, dinnertime has to be a time of enjoyment and relaxation. I used to do so many things while I ate that I had no idea of what I was putting in my mouth. I might have already eaten dinner, but I was ready to eat again.

"Now, I look forward to my meals because I experience them. So much of eating has to do with the way we feel after we eat that the atmosphere is just as important as what we eat. The other night, my husband asked me about a bill that was overdue—and I said, 'That's for later. Right now, I want to concentrate on this steak.' And now, after two months of this, everyone is used to it. I heard my son say to someone on the phone, 'Mom's eating right now,' and I had to smile. It really makes a difference."

Food of the Week

Hey, was that an apple or an apple pie the Snake gave Eve?

Papaya. This tropical fruit has a terrific taste and is a health food as well. A great source of vitamins A and C, it is also loaded with potassium. Peel it, seed it, and cut it into slices to liven up a predictable fruit salad! Even its seeds can be used. They have a tart taste and can be sprinkled into salads or used in sauces.

Applesauce. Applesauce flavored with cranberries or strawberries. You can jazz up homemade applesauce yourself or when you are pressed for time—these are commercially available. "Spiked" applesauce is another way of making a routine fruit dessert memorable. Most important, you will feel satisfied, not deprived. You can enjoy a sweet at the end of a meal without taking in thousands of calories.

Variety Is the Spice of Life—and of Weight Loss

In addition to papaya, your fruit salad can include such treats as kiwis (high in vitamin C and potassium, free of fat and sodium, and its tiny seeds also promote regularity), star fruits, and mangoes (the latter are loaded with vitamins A and C, and are good for the digestion since they contain fiber). Most overweight people stick to the same foods, and the same tastes and flavors, over and over again. But studies have shown that people who eat the largest selection of foods often are the best nourished. By repeating the same meals over and over, you are setting yourself up for a binge. You may *think* that you can "get away with it," but sooner or later the brain gets the message, "I am bored/deprived." So, put that extra energy into "preventive" eating and be adventurous and creative with your fruits and vegetables.

Self-empowerment Exercise for the Week

Take a notebook along with you for the day and jot down every thought you have about yourself, your weight, your fitness level, your willpower, or any thoughts that come up regarding your worth as a person, weight-related or not. When you see a particularly fit-looking or thin person, what are your reactions? Jot them down, too. When someone compliments you or criticizes you, how do you react? Put that in the notebook as well. At the end of the day, you will have a pretty good idea of whether you are sending yourself the right message.

Read over the notes and wherever you come upon a negative, crippling self-message, cross it out and write down one that tells you: *I can do it!*

When you find yourself condemning yourself for a slipup, or when you discover yourself putting yourself down, even though it is "only" in your mind, you know that you are reinforcing a pattern of defeat. What takes place in your mind translates into your reality. It becomes your future, your fate. The term "self-fulfilling prophecy" means a result that *you* have brought about because of your mental attitude.

Sometimes we hypnotize ourselves with so much negativity that we are not even aware of what we are telling ourselves! It becomes a basic attitude that manifests in our body language, in what we are willing to try or are afraid of trying, in whether we reach our goals. The first step is to become aware of what is going on; the second step is to change it. If you use this self-talk notebook honestly, it can become a valuable tool of self-discovery and challenge.

Stress Antidote for the Week

Breathe! Breathe! Breathe!

"The single most effective relaxation technique
I know is conscious regulation of breath."
—Dr. Andrew Weil

You can do this one anywhere, anytime, with anyone watching. Say you are at your mother-in-law's Thanksgiving dinner, and she is pushing a calorie-rich dessert on you. Before replying, try the simple breathing exercise below and you'll feel better (and might even be able to refuse with a smile). Try it in a crowded elevator after a long day at work, in a doctor's office, waiting for test results...instead of grabbing for a bag of pretzels, *breathe.*

What? I already breathe, you say. But no, put your hand on your stomach and feel it flatten as your lungs slowly fill with air—that is, breathe from your belly, not your chest (that is from the diaphragm, the muscle between the chest and abdominal cavity. That's where a baby breathes from, taking deep, steady breaths). Draw the air in through your nostrils. Hold the breath for a count of six. If you can close your eyes for an instant, do so, and picture energy flowing into you with that deep breath. Now breathe out slowly, mildly contracting your stomach muscles. Repeat six to eight times if you have the time, but even once or twice will help. You will feel calmer *immediately*. It is just the technique to use when dealing with a stressful moment at work or at home. Repeated at intervals throughout the day, it gives you little islands of calm in a raging ocean! Let it become a new habit, something you do automatically, without thinking. The way you *used to* nibble and snack.

There are thousands of breathing exercises and all kinds of advanced techniques (expert breathers!) for those who might like to explore this option. *Jumpstart Your Metabolism: How to Lose Weight by Changing the Way You Breathe* by Pam Grout is one such guide. But anyone who decides to take up yoga or research Zen will also pick up valuable breathing techniques. These will produce calming physiological changes, altering the mood and bringing more oxygen into the bloodstream. Trying out a different technique each week would be a great way to start each meeting! Breathe together, as a team!

But even the simple exercise given here will do wonders. "The way we breathe has a profound effect on the way we feel," says psychologist Phil Nuernberger (*Freedom from Stress*). "Many stress-related complaints—whether physical, mental, or emotional—are caused by improper breathing. But fortunately, many of these complaints can be reversed simply by learning to breathe properly." Instead of reaching for a chocolate bar, close your eyes, picture a flower-covered meadow or a snowy mountain and breathe! Practiced regularly, after a period of time you will find yourself automatically breathing deeply for a rush of energy!

Chapter Three: The Meeting

"Every great idea is a simple one."
—Leo Tolstoy

W hat's the most important thing you can do at the meeting? Make it an event! Get people so stirred up that you can be charged with inciting a riot! You and your teammates have endless things to do—chores, responsibilities, and obligations—so the meeting must be, above all, a time of inspiration for everyone. You must be able to show up exhausted and leave with a smile on your face. The meetings should be serious, fun, supportive, memorable, and inspiring! It is the starting point of each week, and the finish line of the last week as well. They are times to take stock of how you've done over the week and to plan new challenges and strategies for the week to come. It doesn't matter if it's you and one other hardy soul or if it's you and three hundred members! The meeting can be a *fiesta,* an island of support and fun in an ocean of demands.

The common denominator of every meeting, from the small, informal one to the large rally, should be the *unexpected.* Your meetings should be a time where you get to try out new things together with your teammates—yoga and belly dancing, bok choy and fencing *(Why not?!),* gardening and garlic, pedicures and pottery—whatever will keep you going! When someone asks you what you're willing to do to get fit and healthy, the answer must be: *anything!*

The meeting is a time to let go of your inhibitions with a raucous, off-key team song or a funny cheer. It's a time to listen to speakers who can inspire and motivate and teach you things you didn't know. For example, M.J. Smith, a speaker at one Dyersville Fight the Fat meeting, taught the members how to make really nutritious, balanced meals in twenty minutes. Five in twenty, that is, five ingredients in twenty minutes (her books are listed in the appendix).

Instead of thinking about the meeting as yet another area in your life where you have to perform—another job, another task, another duty—make it a fun event that will loosen everyone up and get you to look forward to the meetings.

At first you might feel shy about singing team songs and cheers. It will seem so silly! But who cares if it's silly, as long as it works? And trust me, it does work. There's something bonding about *playing* together with your teammates as if you are kids again. Be a child for the night! That's just what you need! It's a way of relieving the grim pressure you put on yourself in this area of weight loss and exercise (and it doesn't matter whether you've tried out ten new diets last year or haven't dieted in the last decade, the pressure is always there).

This kind of release is just what will help you to succeed. If you feel too frantic about anything, you don't deal with it well. You need some distance and some perspective, and nothing gives you that better than laughter.

There was plenty of that at the meetings I attended—everything from giggles and guffaws to good old-fashioned belly laughs. The collective weigh-in was incredible. The "moment of truth" came when each team climbed onto a scale built to weigh semi-trucks loaded with corn or other commodities. The hilarity and laughter and suspense as the members stripped down for the big weigh-in at the Farmers Shipping Association were therapeutic elements of the process. No one felt alone with their problem, trapped by previous failures or by cruel comments and condemnation. Passing a ten foot "fat-o-meter" set up in the middle of town, like weighing in together on a huge scale, was part of the Fight the Fat message: we're in this *together.*

And while in some areas of the U.S.A. it's hard to find a huge truck scale, it's always possible to come up with all kinds of goofy skits and fun ideas to send yourself an important message, one that gets through to you when a so-called more "serious" one won't.

In Monticello, they kicked off their meeting with a skit in which some "nurses" wheeled a stretcher with a very heavy "patient" onto the platform of the school's auditorium. The patient started shouting and gasping, pretending to be in her last agony while a nurse pounded on her chest. Then, suddenly, another nurse reached under the sheets and drew out boxes of cookies and containers of ice cream and candy and the "patient" got up and began doing jumping jacks as the audience went wild. The skit was the first thing on the agenda. It provided a much needed moment of relief at the very beginning, perhaps when it is most needed!

Understanding this principle, Mary Hoeger, Director of Nursing at Mercy Medical Center in Dyersville, combined a serious purpose with a hilarious approach when giving her presentation. As a woman who lost sixty-five pounds, she came onto the platform in a peasant style dress, all browns and plaids and checks, a voluminous dress that covered a very full body shape. She then explained that if her outfit looked special it was because she had bought it for a relative's wedding and she had wanted something different.

"Many of you here know me from the time you or your relatives have been patients in Mercy Medical Center," she announced. "I worked in the cardiac unit at Mercy-Dubuque. I'd lean over my patients and tell them that they needed to lose weight and exercise more. And the beads of sweat were forming on my forehead," she paused. "But of course, they were too polite to answer that I seemed to be having a hard time leaning forward with all my weight! So, I decided that it was time to really do something different!"

Smiling, she started stripping off her dress which, it turned out, was stuck on with Velcro. Underneath—to the amazement of most of the members who had not seen the slow transformation—was the "new" Mary Hoeger, some thirty pounds thinner! "If being a nurse in cardiac doesn't inspire weight loss, what can?" she went on to cheers and applause. She had the crowd in the palm of her hand. That combination of laughter and drama helped make her talk very moving. Everyone was spellbound. It made a big impression.

Another ingredient in the recipe for a good meeting is friendly competition. It's so important to introduce that element of play into our lives! When you're competing with someone else, your attitude changes. Instead of being grimly obsessed with the forty or fifty pounds you have to take off (groan! groan!), suddenly the emphasis shifts to *Let's see who's going to win this week.*

Even if your Fight the Fat team has only five or six members, and even if it's just you and one other friend you've joined forces with, you can put zest into your weight loss with *friendly* competition—note the emphasis. When it's done right, as it was in Dyersville, competition helps you bond with your teammates. You also have fun playing the game! One team had a Better Than Sex Cake delivered to their rivals as a gag (they ended up eating small slivers and giving it away). In Dyersville, rival teams really rooted for each other—it was like competing with yourself. What you heard on all sides in Dyersville was that people were *happy* for the winners. Their achievement pushed the others forward. *If they can do it, so can I!* was the attitude.

Prizes for the winners don't have to be Lincoln Continentals. It's enough just to pick up the winner's lunch tab or to pay for a round of drinks at a bar—provided it's a juice bar. After all, what you're going for is the buzz that comes from rivalry and achievement. In the Dyersville Fight the Fat, there was a grand prize of a makeover—haircut, facial, manicure, pedicure, and massage—for the winner of The Most Body Fat Lost. Like The Most Changed, The Most Body Fat Lost is another effort at shifting the emphasis away from number of pounds lost to where it belongs—on the whole picture. Mercy Medical Center provided the machine to analyze body fat. For your group, it should be easy to get tested at your local hospital. If you prefer you can also frequently find these machines at recreation centers.

Another serious issue that should be made a priority at the meeting is testing blood pressure and cholesterol levels. In Dyersville, volunteers from Mercy administer these tests at the first meeting (lipid profile results are mailed to the members). So, forget the excuse "I just didn't get around to it!" Fight the Fat is about "getting around to it," the "it" being your health and well-being.

In keeping with the serious/wacky rhythm of the Dyersville meeting, such serious stuff was followed by a funny routine dreamed up by a team of Dyersville friends called *Slim Pickens* (they sang a slightly risqué song in very off-key voices, and brought down the house). Then the Mercy nutritionist Jane Clemen took center stage for a short but really helpful talk on nutrition (she explained the food pyramid, a standard tool of nutrition that will be discussed in chapter seven). Not wanting to overload her audience with too many facts or too much advice, she broke up her material into segments, giving a short talk each week.

Without giving it undue importance, another activity that should be included in your meeting is the weekly weigh-in. Have it take place *before* the meeting starts so that nobody goes home discouraged. In Dyersville, the number of pounds each team member has lost is added up to arrive at the grand total (then the teams' totals are added up to see what the town has lost together).

By announcing the collective weight loss, the Fight the Fat organizers are making a statement: you are not alone with that monster called the scale anymore—*What! After working so hard all week, I've only lost a pound! What? After resisting so much temptation, I actually put on a half pound!*—No! You are surrounded with friends who are there to help you through this.

While you're eager to know what you weigh, of course, the scale is probably the *least* important measurement of where you are. *You know this,* but you need to hear it over and over again. Who hasn't gone from a disappointing session with the scale straight to the fridge? Now you have a team to bar that path to the fridge, hold you back, and help you put things in perspective.

Apart from scheduled activities such as weigh-ins and speakers, meetings are also times for members themselves to exchange simple techniques, tricks, methods of coping, and good recipes—whatever comes up. At a meeting I attended, you could see the way that this kind of informal, spontaneous give and take made everyone feel connected. What people had to say didn't matter as much as the fact that they cared enough about one another to say it.

Suzanne, a member of a spin-off Fight the Fat in Monticello thought that this kind of support was crucial (she lost twenty-eight pounds). "I was kind of down in the dumps by week seven. My weight loss had slowed. I was getting so sick of salad that just seeing anything green made me lose my appetite. I mentioned this in passing to Judy, a teammate who loves to cook, and the next week she brought in an excellent suggestion.

"It was a recipe for *Ginger, Green Apple, Sweet Onion, and Coconut Salad* she'd read about in a gourmet magazine, *Food & Wine.* It wasn't only that the suggestion was great—it gave new life to my salad eating that week—but I felt touched that Judy cared enough to copy it out for me. Here's a woman with four kids and a husband who's recovering from a bad car accident, and she takes the time and effort to bring this recipe into the meeting! There was no way I would have let her down by giving up (I had been seriously considering dropping out) even if the recipe had been lousy!

"But it wasn't lousy," she quickly added. "It happens to be a fun recipe that's easy to make. You slice up two Granny Smith apples, one small sweet onion, and one three-inch piece of ginger (which you cut up into ⅛-inch by two-inch matchsticks). Add a half-cup of finely grated, peeled fresh coconut, three tablespoons of shredded basil, three tablespoons of lemon verbena oil, and a little salt and pepper. Mix it up! This amount serves four people. In my case, I ate two portions one day and two the next and that was still okay. I had a good week."

Rhonda, another Monticello member, added, "For me the important thing about exchanging advice is that you tend to put more faith in your teammates' words. Here's someone sitting next to you who you know and who's getting results, so, naturally you want to try out what she's doing, too. For example, a friend of mine told me to use cans as weights (going out and buying weights was just something she wouldn't do, but the cans are right there). She said that usually when you cook in the kitchen, you have to wait for something to boil or defrost and you end up eating. You take a bite of this and a spoonful of that and before you know it, you're down—I guess I should say 'up'—a few hundred calories.

"I listened to her, and now while I wait for things to cook, I take two large cans, tomato cans since they're heavy, and use them like weights. Or I do some stretches. Or, I put the broom behind my neck and over my shoulders to work on my lateral movement—I call it my kitchen gym. I've been keeping to this for a long time now, day after day, and it makes a difference in my morale. Instead of getting demoralized, I start the meal feeling strong, and thinking *yes!*"

In all the meetings I went to, from the big Dyersville rally to the small team get-togethers, you could hear members putting their heads together this way, fitting the pieces of the puzzle in place. There's always an excited buzz of conversation.

For example, you can really get a sense of progress taking place in this conversation overheard after a Dyersville meeting:

Member #1: "Writing down what you eat gives you a handle on what you are doing…For the first few weeks, I didn't do it. I thought, what good does it do? But now I see it makes a difference."

Member #2: "I've been doing real well on my exercises but now I have to start this, too."

Member #3: "I'll do it if you do it."

The meeting is also a good place to let off steam, which is why it's important to establish a no-holds-barred atmosphere. As Fight the Fat team captain Joanne says, "Sometimes people get to feeling discouraged, they get all frustrated and angry and they want to say *screw this!* And that's cool. It's better for them to *talk* about eating than to go out and stuff themselves."

I got the chance to see Joanne in action as team captain at a Tuesday night meeting. As someone who's kept on track through two Fight the Fat campaigns (her total loss: twenty-seven pounds), she had the perfect answer for one of her teammates who announced after the weigh-in: "That's it! I'm out of here! I'm going for a hot fudge Sundae…"

"Try McDonald's," Joanne answered her without missing a beat. "That's where I go when I want one. A hot fudge or hot caramel frozen yogurt sundae—wait a minute—" she took a booklet out of her purse and scanned it. "—will take you about forty-five minutes of power walking to work off."

Now this was not some slick fashion model or weight-loss guru talking. It was a forty-five-year-old mother of two teenage boys whose only exercise for years had been bringing the family's groceries in from the supermarket! She is a woman who has taken off twenty-eight pounds and who looks *good* and who now goes mountain biking with her husband every Sunday. Her teammates could relate to her. They could see themselves achieving the success she had so they listened to her…they *really* listened.

Each meeting should start with a *bang,* and each meeting should close with a memorable final thought, some vivid message that lingers after everyone goes home. It can be a quote that got to you, a story, or a meaningful memory. One Dyersville team—we'll call them the *Nevermore Fat* since they want to remain anonymous—had a different member close the meeting each week, giving everyone a chance to do some serious thinking, and to take some time preparing for what they would say. They asked each member to explain why Fight the Fat was important to them.

At one meeting, a woman who was thirty-something pounds overweight started off by saying that although she hadn't lost many pounds *yet* (her emphasis), during Fight the Fat she had stopped gaining, and she had come to see this as a victory.

"When I was five or six," she went on, speaking in a low but confident voice. "I wouldn't let my parents photograph me without an ice cream cone in one hand and a bag of candy in the other. That's how important food was to me. By the time I was in fifth grade, I weighed one hundred and seventy pounds. My parents pushed food on me and then they blamed me because I was fat. For some of us, what we have to fight is a lifelong brainwashing. *Eat something, you'll feel better,* and it's very hard to break this kind of training.

"Now my two kids also have a weight problem, and when I talk to them about it, they are like, *Mom, why can't you just love us the way we are?* I try to explain to them that if it wasn't a matter of their health, I wouldn't care—but they don't go for that.

"That's why I want to change. I want to show them that I value the life God gave me. When my kids see me sweating and doing push-ups against the wall, they say, *'Hey! Get a load of Mom!'* They know I'm for real!"

Your Workbook

The Bulletin Board

For those who have lost weight (countless times) and gained it back, these favorite quotes from Fight the Fat members will be heartening.

"Success is not purchased at any one time, but on the installment plan."
—Joan

"The first time you tried to walk, you fell down! But you didn't give up, did you? Failure is just the first step on the road to success. You may have had this or that setback. All right! Now you know what doesn't work."
—Sally

"Your IQ is not nearly as important as your will!"
—Robert

"If I'm not free to fail, I'm not free to take risks, and everything in life that's worth doing involves a willingness to risk failure. Although I have had thirty books published, there are at least six unpublished books that have failed, but which have been necessary for the book that then gets published. The same thing is true in all human relationships. Unless I'm willing to open myself up to risk and to being hurt, then I'm closing myself off to love and friendship."
—Madeline L'Engle, author of *A Wrinkle in Time*

"I play to win even when common sense should tell me that I no longer have a chance. Even when I have been playing at my worst, or when all the breaks have been going against me, I approach each new day, each new hole, as a glorious opportunity to get going again."
—Arnold Palmer, professional golfer

If You Need to Be Scared!

- Obesity is second only to smoking as the leading cause of preventable death.
- The rising rate in diabetes in young people, even children, matches the ever-rising rate of obesity.
- Type 2 diabetes, *which is more likely to occur among the overweight,* if caught early, can be controlled through a simple combination of exercise, change in diet, and weight loss. If ignored, it can lead to a serious condition requiring lifelong medication.

Your Journal

Hey, you've got to bounce back if you want to survive!

"Our greatest glory is not in always succeeding,
but in rising up every time we fail."
— Ralph Waldo Emerson

Think about that—it's as true today as when Emerson said it a hundred years ago. For your journal this week, remember a situation in which you failed to achieve a goal you had set for yourself (it can be, but it doesn't have to be, weight related). Analyze the way you reacted to such a failure.

1) *Did you "beat yourself up" for it? What kind of self-talk went on? After failing, did you try to set another, more realistic goal? Or did you give up completely?*

2) *Now, in the perspective time brings, do you see ways in which could you have handled the situation differently? What are they?*

3) *Are you the kind of person who learns from the past? List at least three things that your past mistakes have taught you.*

These last questions are perhaps the most important:

1) *How did your success/failure affect your self-esteem?*
2) *Are you the kind of person who can bounce back from failures? Or, do setbacks leave you wallowing in despair?*
3) *What are steps that you can take to break this pattern?*

Bringing these questions up with your teammates for general discussion would give your next meeting a significant focus.

Healthy Habit for the Week

Discovery of the century:
I'm not hungry! I'm cold!
I'm not hungry, I just *feel deprived!*

You're going to like this one! No, we're not going to tell you run up and down a mountain before every meal. We're going to make a suggestion that you will *enjoy*, one that requires *zero* willpower, and yet is a key both to losing weight and to keeping it off!

Studies have shown that people who *regularly* include soups in their diet have better control over their eating patterns and maintain that control over long periods of time (*regularly*—that is, we're talking frequently, almost every day here).

The body tells the brain *we're getting a lot of nourishment.* There is something satisfying about delicious, hot soup. Plus, it takes a long time to finish a bowl, spoonful by spoonful. It's a great way to get your vegetables (bulky) and some soups (like vegetable soups without sugar) are virtually unlimited in their possibilities. The following are some suggestions. *So, soup it up!*

An all-purpose, throw-it-in-and-let-it-boil, starter-off soup might be for you. You can put almost anything in this one *except* the kids' galoshes.

I'll tell it to you the way it was told to me on the run by a woman who's a really healthy cook. "Experiment!" she cried. "I always fool around even with gourmet recipes until I get exactly the taste I like! With vegetable soup, I just keep throwing in everything I can think of, from carrots and onions to every type of leafy greens...cabbage, shredded...garlic and celery...mustard greens make a really healthy addition, as do collards. Water to cover, sometimes I add some vegetable bouillon and *herbs!* Thyme, oregano, sage, parsley, ginger (a particular strong flavor). If you want to sneak in a potato, you'll still have a practically "free" soup (calorie free, that is).

"If you have time, also, it's a nice idea to sauté some onions and mushrooms in a wok first (I like woks for this purpose and for stir-frys. Since they have more surface area for frying, there's less chance of your food burning and all you need is a little bit of oil)."

Here is a soup idea from *The New American Diet Cookbook* by Sonja L. Connor and William E. Connor.

Black Bean Soup
⅛ cup (10 pieces) sun-dried tomatoes (not packed in oil)
1 cup boiling water
1 to 2 cups finely chopped onion
3 cloves garlic, minced
¼ to ½ tsp cayenne pepper or 1 tsp Tabasco sauce to taste
1 tbsp. vegetable oil
1 tsp cumin
1 tsp (or less) light salt
2 cans unsalted diced tomatoes
2 15-ounce cans black beans, not drained
¼ cup chopped fresh cilantro
Nonfat yogurt or nonfat sour cream, for garnish

1) In a small bowl, cover the sun-dried tomatoes with 1 cup boiling water and set aside.

2) In a soup pot, sauté the onions, garlic, and cayenne in the oil for five minutes, stirring frequently until the onions are translucent.

3) Add the cumin, light salt, tomatoes (including the liquid), and black beans.

4) Bring to a boil; reduce the heat to low and cover.

5) Simmer for 20 minutes, stirring occasionally to prevent sticking.

6) Drain and chop the softened sun-dried tomatoes. Add them to the soup and cook 10 minutes.

7) Stir in the cilantro and remove the soup from the heat.

8) Purée half of the soup in a blender or food processor and return it to the pot. If the soup is too thick, add water.

9) Heat the soup and serve with a dollop of yogurt or sour cream. Serves eight.

(110 calories, 2 grams fat)

If you add a plate of brown rice as a side dish along with the Black Bean Soup, you get a "complete protein"—more protein than steak, a low-fat energy booster.

Reward for the Week

SHHH! Don't tell anyone, but give yourself a three-day weekend (you deserve it!). In addition to President's Day and Veteran's Day and Memorial Day Weekend, there is now Fight the Fat weekend just for you! Your boss won't like it, but give yourself one day off for your health—your mental health—as a reward for having come so far. Make it a way of celebrating Week Three!

Use it just for yourself. A walk, a long talk with a friend, a trip (after all, you have three days!) to a magnificent old mansion or a historical site or to the ocean or mountains. Let no one and nothing disturb you on this day. It is a present from you to you!

Team Activity for the Week

Massage: what a dynamic way to bond with your teammates! There's nothing more basic than our sense of touch! When you go to other cultures where virtual strangers hug you or put their arms around your waist, you realize how uptight our society is about people touching each other in a friendly, non-sexual way. Yet touch is so basic to the way we relate to each other! What's more comforting than a gentle squeeze at the back of the neck from a friend? Isn't that how we reassure kids? And aren't kids always putting their arms around you?

We can't change the culture overnight, but we can show and receive more affection from people we trust. And massage is another way of using our sense of touch for comfort.

Sally, a Fight the Fat member who lost more than twenty-four pounds, swears by it: "My husband wouldn't join the class with me. He said '*I don't go for all that 'touchy feely' stuff!*' I said, 'Okay! Stay home and fix the lawnmower! There are plenty of teammates who want to come to class with me!' Now he *loves* it when I try out my techniques on him—knuckles, elbows, a back-walk*, the works. And though he can't match me, I've taught him some good moves of his own. If a teammate hadn't pushed me on, though, I never would have started. Now massage is a major part of my life. There's nothing I look forward to more at the end of a long, hard day."

(*Caution: *only* do the back-walk when you've learned from a pro how to do it right.)

Whether you pay a professional masseur or masseuse or you take classes and swap massages with your fellow students, massage is a great way of getting in touch with your body. For so many overweight people, their bodies have become just these *huge burdens* they have to drag from one place to another. Massage reminds you of the poem that your body is! (As the psalmist says: "I will praise You for I am wonderfully made!")

You can find massage workshops in yoga schools and continuing education programs. There are also usually local massage training centers.

For those who are given to "comfort eating"—food as a security blanket—a comfort massage is a good substitute. When we were kids, we were stroked when we were upset or even just as a mark of affection. That's why a good massage can trigger the positive feelings we associated with this kind of petting. To begin, all you need is a jar of massage oil and a few simple "moves" like the ones given below. When you get more advanced, there's a whole "massage world" out there with all kinds of extras such as massage rollers, massage stones, massage tables, acupressure, body massagers, and scented oils! Sandalwood, patchouli, jasmine, and rose are really sensual—or mix your own scent using an essence and unscented massage oil.

Recommended for massage: either silence or soft music. Talk keeps the mind active and massage is meant to relax and relieve pressure and tension. Become jelly!

In addition to the following simple massage moves, the key to a great massage is to *improvise!* When you and your massage partner know each other better, you will get an increased sense of what the other needs.

Pressing: press gently with your fingertips across your partner's forehead, down along the nose, and around the cheekbones and jawbone. (Be careful around the eyes.) Then massage your partner's earlobes.

You can release tension in less sensitive places like the arms and thighs and calves by making fists and pressing your knuckles into the muscles. Keep moving your knuckles in smooth movements. Repeat six to seven times.

Palming: put your open hands palm down on your partner's skin and move in a stroking motion. Very calming (plus it warms up the skin and prepares it for kneading).

Kneading: that's what we do when we're making bread. For massage purposes, your partner has to become a lump of dough! Put your palm on your partner's shoulder or back to start with, sticking out your thumb and making semi-circles or half moons with it. At the same time, gently press the fingertips of your other hand into the skin from the other side of the semi-circle (you'll be creating the sensation of a gentle pinch). Repeat several times, moving along the body. (Suggestions contributed by Ralph Kramer, physical therapist and masseur.)

There are many different kinds of massage, from Swedish to Shiatsu, and you may want to experiment with a few until you find one that suits your needs. Although some people enjoy being kneaded like a ball of dough, deep massage does not necessarily mean the application of a great deal of force: a skilled masseur or masseuse can release tension and relax the muscles by gently touching pressure points in just the right sequence.

Gina, a masseuse who often works with overweight clients, remarked that it is not unusual for her clients to begin to cry in the middle of a massage. "They are carrying around so much stress and tension without knowing it. And then they start to cry—literally from relief. My treatments provide a much needed catharsis for them and I can *feel* the difference after a few sessions. I can feel how much more flexible their muscles are. So much has been bottled up inside that they have let go of."

Golden Rule for the Week

Some "Do's and Don'ts" in the Looking-Ahead Department

It's all about looking ahead! If you're facing the weekend with an empty fridge, or with one packed with treats for the kids and nothing for yourself, you don't have to be a swami to predict disaster. Part of what healthy weight loss entails is *paying attention. Focus.* It's not about starvation but about *what will I eat next?*

Don't wait until it's the middle of the afternoon and everyone in the office is taking a coffee break (make that a chocolate croissant break). Don't wait until you get home at the end of a day of stress and strain and are starving. That's when your willpower is at its lowest and you are not likely to make the best choices. That is, you'll eat enough to feed a third world village for a year! Prepare healthy, low-calorie, and *delicious* snacks you can take along with you to work. And have something *special* waiting that can take the edge off your hunger when you get home so that you're not snacking on junk while getting dinner ready.

Sliced, peeled carrots are not going to do it when you're saying *no!* to sugar-frosted doughnuts. Now, if you mix some diced carrots, or mash some boiled ones, with a little pineapple, a handful of raisins, some shredded apple, and a fresh lime or lemon, hmmm, sounds interesting! How about a grilled banana or pineapple mixed together with low-fat yogurt? You get the idea. Mix it, dice it, core it, and peel it. Use your imagination to give the bulk of unlimited carrots some sweetness and deliciosity! You'll have your fellow office workers salivating and looking at your carrots with envious eyes!

You can do this with any unlimited guilt-free veggie. All it takes is—yes, you said it—*preparation!* If a good breakfast takes time to prepare, have it all ready and waiting to be heated up the night before. As Fran, a physical therapist who lost thirty pounds since joining Fight the Fat says, "If you're on your way to a stress-producing event like a visit with some relatives you just can't stand, have low-fat treats in the car to fortify you before and afterwards! I used to end up losing control and stuffing myself every time I visited my husband's sister. Now I know I have an all fruit and yogurt smoothie waiting for me on the counter the minute I walk through my front door, and boy does that help!"

This kind of preparation equals commitment. If you spend fifty dollars on vegetables and fruits for the weekend, you will think twice before throwing away all that money by bingeing on ice cream! You've put too much time and effort into shopping for veggies! That's just the way the mind works—so take advantage of it. Remember: winning a battle is all about strategy. You don't have to be a Boy Scout to adopt their motto: *Be Prepared!*

Food of the Week

Broccoli. So you hate broccoli! So what! Just *disguise* it. Shred it, grill it, stir-fry it with your favorite fish or meat, a teaspoon of sesame oil, ginger to taste, and a clove of garlic. You'll forget it's even in the pan. Make broccoli slaw for God's sake! That's coleslaw with broccoli shredded in. Broccoli can have more disguises than Mata Hari.

Why should I bother? For starters, it's a great source of carotene and vitamin C. As if that's not enough, it *also* delivers plenty of calcium—we're talking strong bones and teeth here. Broccoli also contains *indoles,* which fight cancer. Look for firm stems and a deep rich green when you're buying it (reject stalks that are yellowing). If you're not a broccoli lover, then just chop it up in a well-seasoned macaroni salad or serve it in vegetable soup.

If you copy this paragraph out and paste it up on your fridge, I guarantee that you will end up eating broccoli at least once a week. It's hard to ignore such a great gift of health at such a low price! Okay, it's not chocolate, but can chocolate do all of the above for you? Get smart, kiddo!

Chickpeas are sometimes known as garbanzo beans or ceci. If you mash them up they are called humus, a tasty Mid-Eastern sauce used to liven up all kinds of dishes from vegetables and rice to meat. "One of my team's challenges was 'Try a food you've never had before. But make sure it's a healthy one,'" says Suzanne of the Dubuque Fight the Fat. "So, I went to a health food store and ended up bringing a lot of stuff home. Some of it I wasn't all that crazy about, but the humus was great—better than a cheese dip I always used to buy (and healthy, too).

"When I first showed up at work with my emergency pack," adds Suzanne, "everyone was curious. And when I unpacked a container with cucumbers, carrots, celery, and a jar of humus, my friends said '*You've got to be kidding!*' But I just said '*Taste it!*'"

Suzanne's humus is more than a garnish for her vegetables. It's also a great source of protein, fiber, iron, potassium, *and* the B vitamins, thiamin and niacin. What a difference from the "empty" calories (empty nutritionally) of Suzanne's old mid-morning snack of chocolate chip cookies.

Her total weight loss so far?

"I don't like to think about it that way anymore," Suzanne said. "I don't think about *weight loss*, I think about *health gain*. But if you have to know, I'll just say that I'm wearing something I couldn't get into for years."

Self-empowerment Exercise for the Week

Creative Visualization

Imagining the new you. The imagination lets us *see* the reality we are striving to create. You can buy tapes and books (see appendix) devoted completely to this fascinating subject. To begin with, you might want to rely on their guidance for the images you focus on. Or you might want to imagine in detail some triumphant or supremely happy moment in your life and "hold on to it" every day.

Take time every day to visualize yourself after you have become the new healthy you. Picture yourself springing up from your chair or jogging through the woods in spring. Perhaps you have photos from a time when you were more active/fit—put them up where you will see them every day. All kinds of photos can be used for the visualization exercise since you glance at them—with or without concentrating—countless times during a day. You keep taking in their message.

One Fight the Fat member kept a photo on the kitchen wall of a total stranger—a woman who had jogged by on the road when she happened to be taking pictures of her garden. "I like this woman *so much* because she is not a professional model. She does not look perfect. She is out of breath and even a little overweight, but she's sticking to it. Look at that grin on her face. It says to me, *I'm going to make it.* I keep her up there on my wall for inspiration." By concentrating on images of ourselves as we would like to be, we close the gap between what *is* and *what will be*.

Two interesting books on the subject are *Getting Well Again* by Carl Simonton, Matthew Simonton, and James Creighton, and *Healing Yourself:*

A Step-by-Step Program for Better Health Through Imagery by Martin L. Rossman, M.D.

Stress Antidote for the Week

Try this one out every day for a week and see how it will change both the way you feel and the way you look at things:

Pick out a beautiful place that you love to be. If you are in the city, it might be a botanical garden or a promenade near a river or a boardwalk near the ocean; in the country it might be a quiet valley, a long field, or an orchard. Allow yourself to enjoy what is before you. When stray thoughts, worries, angers, or fears come to mind *let go of them.* Thoughts will come and go but after a while the special quality of the place will take over. Most of us rush through life and don't give ourselves the chance to receive the strength and serenity that is before us in nature. I tried this exercise in a part of Prospect Park in Brooklyn that I thought I knew very well. But when I returned week after week, so many details of the place became vivid that I had never noticed before; the small changes seemed dramatic—the spirit of the place spoke to me.

"Climb the mountains and get their good tidings.
Nature's peace will flow into you as sunshine flows into trees.
The winds will blow their own freshness into you, and the storms
their energy, while cares will drop off like autumn leaves."
— John Muir

Chapter Four: Stress

"For fast acting relief, try *slowing down*."
—Lily Tomlin

"Half our life is spent trying to find something to do with the time we have rushed through life trying to save."
—Will Rogers

Now you have a team, even if it's only one Fight the Fat partner, to help you come to terms with stress, your patterns, and the way it relates to your eating. In short, your MO. In this area, a teammate can be helpful because it's as hard to be objective about your mental attitude as it is to give yourself a haircut. Your teammate is your mirror. So, when considering the following issues, do so with your teammate. That can finally be the piece of the puzzle that was missing.

Stress

Do you really, secretly, love it? This may sound ridiculous at first, but many people are *stress junkies*. They use stress as a way of getting things done, a fuel to keep them going. They use it to fend off depression and lethargy. It gives them a buzz. It makes them feel "alive."

It's a drug they've gotten hooked on without even realizing it. They need their "stress" fix and then they need their "food" fix to help them cope with the stress! It's a pattern that they've chosen, even if they're not aware of it. For them, stress and pressure have become the norm, a way of life.

What, me? Yes, you! Try working on these questions with your teammates (your teammates will keep you honest):

1) *What are three reasons for stress in my life?*
2) *What are three ways I could turn these around?*

3) *What are three reasons I don't want to?*

4) *Where would I be without my stress?*

(For more stress exercises, see the Workbook for this chapter.)

Take Jennifer, a Fight the Fat member who works for a lawyer in Dubuque. A single mother with three young children, she had knocked off more than twenty pounds after coming to terms with just one stress factor in her life.

"My mornings used to be crazy for me," Jennifer told me, doing the walk as she talked the talk—that is, working out on her treadmill. "I work for a lawyer who comes in late. An important part of my job is to be there on time and if I'm not there at nine o'clock I'm fired. That's practically what my boss said when he hired me, and it comes down to that. I have to open up the office, let clients in, and take calls while getting things ready for the day. And I kept just barely getting there on time...before work I'd be busy getting the kids up, pushing them to get dressed and through breakfast, and then dropping them off at school (all the while grabbing muffins or danishes for myself).

"That was the routine. On the way to work, I'd always be drinking coffee and finishing off a second or sometimes even a third danish [this is by nine A.M.].

"There was no way I could handle all the pressure every morning without at least one danish (if I tried to go without one, I would feel like crying). When I couldn't get into my biggest size dress anymore, I joined Fight the Fat. That was a real turning point for me.

"My teammates were great. They've saved me. We've saved each other so many times in the last three years. Just having someone to confide in makes such a difference. I've been through so much with them that they've become family. Every Saturday morning we walk or work out, and then we go down to a little place called Lorna's Kitchen and we chat and have coffee with muffins and talk to each other about our problems.

"So," she added, "I listened when a teammate said to me, *Jennifer, you've just got to get up earlier. You've got to give yourself time to breathe and relax and come to yourself before work!*

"I tried it and she was right. Now I go to sleep earlier and wake up earlier and do everything more slowly. And because I get to work *early* I have plenty of time to prepare for the new day.

"I do some stretches; I write in my journal; I always make sure I have a healthy breakfast that I bring with me and that I eat *slowly*. I feel like a different person now. I have more self-respect. Now when I look back at the old me clutching those danishes as I drove to work, I can see how desperately I needed to change."

Stress and Bingeing

When Fight the Fat organizers asked members what set them off on their last binge, these were some of the answers:

- My son got sick on a day when I had an important meeting and my backup didn't answer her phone.
- The dentist told me I needed a root canal.
- I bounced a check and it screwed up my credit.
- I'm divorced and I was invited to a family affair, and I hate to go alone.
- My car died.
- My mother-in-law always criticizes me.
- My husband doesn't like the way I look.

The list went on, but you get the picture. "People don't [necessarily] eat because they're hungry. They eat because they're stressed out," concludes Fight the Fat organizer Dianna Kirkwood. "That's the No. 1 reason I hear all the time!"

If you stop to think about that, it's pretty amazing. Hunger, a basic instinct, can have very little to do with it.

"And I understand why this is so," Dianna continued, "I'm a stress-eater myself. In the modern world, the clock keeps ticking. You always have a thousand things to do and no time to do it. So we eat."

"Bottom line," says Freda, an energetic team captain from Monticello who came very close to a stroke because of high blood pressure, "is if you eat to calm down, you're a stress-eater. The reason doesn't matter."

"I try to get rid of stress by walking it off," Rosie, a Fight the Fat success story (thirty-four pounds lost over a two-year period) says at a team meeting where the members brainstorm. "But sometimes I still *need* to eat when I'm upset. Only now I have a lot of healthy stuff around. I fill up with lots of salad which I *drown* in different low-calorie dressings I've experimented with (I've made up some of them myself). Or, I start to bake bread. That's very soothing I've discovered."

"Bread?" another member asks with surprise.

"If you want," Rosie offers, "we can bake bread together at my place next meeting. The bread machine makes it a cinch; but I only use it when I'm pressed for time. I like to knead it and let it set and knead it again...It's not an instant process. You have to let it rise three times and the smell of baking fills the whole house. Bread you buy in stores is a husk of what bread used to be. By the time the bread is ready, it makes me feel better no matter what's bothering me."

"But don't you end up eating the whole loaf?" someone asked.

"There's something so satisfying about the whole process that I usually don't. Also, you can make a small loaf. But if I feel like eating more of it, it's okay," Rosie answered. "I can always exercise it off. And the bread you bake is really healthy. There's a lot of protein in the wheat germ and you don't bleach out vitamins and things like that! It's a big difference from filling up on junk food."

Rosie's suggestion triggers others, and by the time the meeting is over, a list of "foods to eat in an emergency" is compiled. One great recipe for "healthy fries" is given in the Workbook section (in the Healthy Habit of the Week). The point is that if you *have to* turn to food in an emergency, you can do it. Only do it in a way that isn't self-destructive—and combine the food with other calming techniques such as exercise.

A Fight the Fat slogan goes this way: *It's not what happens to us, but the way we react to it!* Which is why when it comes to stress, *Attitude is everything!*

As Fight the Fat organizer Dianna Kirkwood said during an interview, "I wish I could write these words a hundred feet high to impress them on you. I wish I could put it on the wrapper of every Ding Dong and bag of potato chips. Make these three words your mantra. They will keep you going! When you get angry and discouraged, when you are ready to give up and give in, repeat these words like a prayer—*Attitude is everything!* Write it on your notepad in the office, on your fridge, on your checkbook, and license plates. These three words can make you thin and fit!

"Make your attitude better, and you will improve not only the shape of your body, but your entire life (those pounds are just a symptom that your life patterns need work!)."

> "You must accept the cards dealt by life.
> But it is up to *you* to decide how to play them."
> — Voltaire

One large source of discomfort that comes under the category *unavoidable stress* is economic—paying the bills—a huge source of stress for Fight the Fat members. If you think that living in a small town in Iowa is less stressful than working for a law firm in New York City, think again! The image of a relaxed life in rural America is a myth. Jobs, families, and community commitments are just as demanding there. As one team captain ("No names, please!") who will remain anonymous said: "Many of the members of our group are farmers or farm wives. My husband is in construction—but when the farmers hurt, everyone else around here feels it. The last two years, the dairy prices have been bad. And the pigs, they're gone. There are hardly any hogs now because of the large confinement centers, and this used to be the hog capital of the world! Many of the smaller farmers have [been] pushed out of the business and that leads to a lot of stress. Many farms have gone under in recent years and the farmers are finding work in other places as carpenters, truck drivers, and so on. And we're talking about family farms, farms that have been passed on for generations. There is a tremendous amount of stress and pressure here from that."

Another anonymous Fight the Fat member said, "My husband lost our dairy farm two years ago. Now he works in maintenance for the nursing home and has a second job in the lumber yard. At first it was hard for him—hard on his pride—plus we had to adjust to a whole new life. We both were overweight and the doctor told my husband that it was affecting his heart. He also has diabetes in his family. My daughter, who joined Fight the Fat, said, 'You lost the farm and you can't do anything about that. But both of you can do something about your weight. If you join, Dad will join. You don't want him getting sick on top of everything.' She convinced us that it was time to think about what we could do for our health."

Fight the Fat gave these people a new focus. It made them think about power walking and nutrition instead of dwelling on what they had lost. It gave them positive goals that they could accomplish with some effort. It gave them a boost.

Stacey, a dedicated Fight the Fat member, had this to add on the subject: "Oh, I know that I eat from stress. I lost my mom five years ago and I lost my dad just recently. It makes a big difference in your life when you go through these things. It is strange how stress affects you because, you know, I've had it both ways. I've been so upset I couldn't eat a thing. And then I've been in states where I could do nothing but eat.

"When my mom was diagnosed with cancer, we spent seven weeks with her. I come from a family of six and we all took turns spending the night. My mom didn't want to be alone. She was scared, so we always stayed with her in twos. It was a very hard time. All my normal patterns were thrown off. I couldn't prepare my own foods. I had to eat whatever was available in the hospital. My sleep was broken up. But I really only started bingeing later, after it was all over."

That is another way that stress affects people: *delayed stress syndrome.* You manage well during the crisis, but when it's all over, you pay the price. After two days of what she called "Crazy eating. Eating everything in sight," she wanted to stop. The months of hard work she had put in with her team, and all the effort, paid off. This out-of-control eating was now the exception in her life, not the rule. She *missed* her morning walk. She *missed* her large salad. She *looked forward* to her next team meeting. In the end, her friends on the team gave her more comfort than the ice cream and cake she used to turn to. She was no longer the same person she had been before she joined Fight the Fat. A healthy lifestyle had grown on her.

You start eating because you're stressed and then the eating itself becomes a source of stress. It's a vicious cycle.

In every case where members formed good relationships with a team member, they said that talking things out with their teammates was a big stress reducer. Of course, the sources of stress were different for everyone. What stresses out one person won't affect another. But the common denominator for stress-eaters is that pressure, anger, grief, or even just sheer exhaustion sends a message to the brain: "Eat! You'll feel better."

In addition to empathy, team members can "pool" their interests and hobbies as a way of stress fighting. For example, Joyce, of the Dyersville Hardee's team *Starlites,* turns to quilting when she feels stress getting to be too much for her. Although she loves to walk, Joyce needed something special besides. When the kids come over (her children are grown) and she starts baking their favorite cakes and treats, she has a terrific way of diverting her attention from food. Her quilts have won prizes (Best of Show at the Iowa State Fair) and she's been offered money for them, but she loves them too much to sell them. Quilting has given her a wonderfully creative outlet for her energy.

Another one of Joyce's teammates, who sings in the church choir, talked about how it strengthened her. "The words, [and] the hymns you're singing are *uppers*. Getting together with a group of people you like to work on something you care about with makes a lot of difference." Still another member invited her teammates to join a Birdathon sponsored by the Audubon society (www.audubon.org/bird/birdathon).

"Once you get into bird watching, you can't imagine how much joy and peace it will give you! The sudden flashes of color, [and] the bird songs really enrich your life."

If you live in a place like Dyersville, Iowa, (where, by the way, the bald eagle is making a come back) so much the better. But even if you live in a place like New York City, a simple thirty-minute subway ride to Queens will take you to a marshy Audubon bird preserve!

A benefit of teaming up with coworkers is that most firms have a stake in promoting their employees' health. Some companies (and their health providers) will offer incentives to employees to join Fight the Fat, such as refunding the membership fee upon completion of the ten weeks. Others will sponsor speakers, provide on-site fitness opportunities, or other support—and this is true whether it's an organization like Mercy Medical Center in Dyersville or the Dyersville McDonald's with its *Big Macs* team, made up of employees.

On a more personal level, says Leah, just having your coworkers rooting for you is great. "You turn on your computer and there's a *flash* from a team member: *Try chilled papaya. It's delicious.* Or there will be a little message, *Come on! You've got what it takes!* When I had a really rough month and started eating in my old way, someone—to this day I don't know who—put a "health pack" on my desk (fruit, low-fat snacks, and even a soothing tape to listen to in my car!). Together with the pack there was this note, *So you've messed up a little! So what! Let's get back on track together. Come to the exercise session tonight, even if you only end up doing a single set of sit-ups or push-ups! We can do it! We will be fit!* I didn't go back that night, but I did the next week. And I've been going ever since."

While these "at work" teams were very successful, some people preferred a different team dynamic. One team in Cascade is made up of acquaintances (who became close friends *after* joining) and who "swore each other to secrecy to discuss personal problems."

But in the long run, it doesn't matter whether the team focuses on emotional issues, or whether, like Leah's office team, it makes stretching and healthy recipes the main agenda. These are personal preferences.

What matters is being on a team. Period.

Every time you go to a team meeting, the message you are giving yourself is *These people have the same problem I do and together we can overcome it.* It is a message that automatically lowers your stress level. Every time you call up a teammate or get a call from one you are telling yourself *I am not alone.*

"What stresses me out?" asks Joanne, twenty-seven pounds lighter from Fight the Fat. "The answer to that used to be *everything*. My new answer is—*Whatever I let stress me out.* My teammates and I have learned that it's up to us."

Your Workbook

Exercises, Questions, Tips, & Points to Ponder for Week 4 of Fight the Fat

---

The Bulletin Board

Among the thoughts for your bulletin board this week, this one especially applies to the *stress factor*:

"We can never be really prepared for that which is wholly new.
We have to adjust ourselves, and every radical adjustment is a crisis in self-esteem; we undergo a test, we have to prove ourselves. It needs great self-confidence to face drastic change without inner trembling."
—Eric Hoffer, longshoreman and writer

"It's hard to beat a person who never gives up."
—Babe Ruth

"Success is living up to your potential. That's all. Wake up with a smile and go after life. Don't just show up at the game or office. Live it, enjoy it, taste it, smell it, feel it."
—Joe Kapp, football player and coach

"The deeds you do today are the only sermon some people will hear today."
—St. Francis of Assisi

"Happiness in this world, when it comes, comes incidentally. Make it the object of pursuit, and it leads us on a wild-goose chase, and is never attained. Follow some other object, and very possibly we may find that we have caught happiness without dreaming of it."
—Nathaniel Hawthorne

"It's not the same to talk of bulls as to be in the bull ring!"
—Rita, Fight the Fat member

Your Journal

Challenge: *live one day at a time and make it a masterpiece.* What can you do to carry out this advice today, right now, at this moment? Fight the Fat member Melissa "weighed in" with this suggestion. "When my team captain read this challenge during the meeting, I thought about it and decided to call a sister I had not spoken to for the last seven years—we had a bad fight over nonsense when my mother died. As soon as the meeting finished, I got on the phone and told her that I missed her and we cried and made up. I felt as if a weight had been lifted from my chest. I didn't realize I was carrying around so much anger and upset. And it helped me with the program, too. I felt so good from what I had done! I realized that if I hadn't been trying to get my life under control with Fight the Fat, I probably would have just eaten my way through that day. Instead I really can say it was a masterpiece."

Making the day a masterpiece can mean forgiving someone—it can mean going to a concert, stopping yourself at the beginning of a binge, taking a long walk, or just feeding the birds! What will your choice be?

Healthy Habit for the Week

Prepare an old favorite—in a healthy way. After a while, your taste buds adjust. If you're used to having ice cream, begin going for frozen low-fat yogurt! Or, if ice cream is a must for you, try a low-fat, low-calorie brand. *Some of the low-fat brands can be even higher than ice cream calorie-wise—watch out!* Look for fat *and* calorie "bargains" like:

- Dole Whip, four ounces: 70 calories, 1 gram fat
- Sweet 'n' Low, four ounces: 80 calories, 2 grams fat
- Sherbet, four ounces: 135 calories, 2 grams fat

- A graham cracker topped with a teaspoon or two of peanut butter and half of a banana won't equal banana cream pie...right away. But as time goes by, it will do the trick.

Here is one good example of a way we can eat and still Fight the Fat (contributed by Fight the Fat member Leah who loves to eat potatoes but who loves her body more!).

Leah's Fight the Fat Fries

This one is really easy. Instead of filling up on artery-clogging fries, try slicing one or even two potatoes very thin. In a Pam-coated pan or on a sheet of aluminum foil coated with Pam, put the sliced potatoes in a toaster oven or a regular oven at 350°. Sprinkle with paprika and spices to taste and bake for about a half-hour. If you need a teaspoon of olive oil to sprinkle over your Fight the Fat chips, it won't kill you—in fact, if you get used to looking forward to *this kind of treat*, you have made a giant step forward toward the new thinner and healthier you.

Reward for the Week

Give yourself a complete makeover—the works—from a facial to a pedicure. For the men, get to a pool and go for a leisurely swim followed by a rubdown and/or sauna. The idea is to come out feeling *good* at a calorie price of *zero* while learning to experience your body in a positive way. Enjoy the process of taking care of your appearance and taking care of your body, no matter what your weight is.

Choose a day for your makeover when you have time. There's a reason why hairdressers are great talkers: that trip to the beauty salon can be a tension-reliever, a time to relax, maybe to gab and joke. Make it a habit! You will look forward to your makeover day the way you used to look forward to that hot fudge sundae. The more non-food techniques you have of giving to yourself, the better. As Rebecca Radcliffe writes in *Enlightened*

Eating, "A person is set up to develop an addiction if [they have] only one way to deal with the stresses in [their] life. Overuse of any single coping strategy becomes addictive."

Team Activity for the Week

In keeping with the issue of the week, do these stress exercises together with your teammates. Together, you can clarify what you need to work on in this area of your life.

Step 1 in Stress Reduction Is Awareness

Figure it out—together. Go through a typical day in your life and decide when and where you are suffering from too much stress. Remember: an overburdened morning can result in out-of-control eating *later on,* during the nighttime. Daily exchanges with a hostile or nasty person (especially one given to making cracks about your weight) can also result in delayed eating. Consider these questions:

1) *Long-term solutions?*
2) *Short-term solutions?*
3) *What healthy (healthier) foods can I use for times when I need to eat?*
4) *What are some activities I can use to reduce stress?*
5) *Team Focus Questions. How can we tackle the stress problem as a team? What kinds of creative team plans can we come up with that will be stress-reducers?*

Avoidable versus Unavoidable Stress

1) *How much of my stress comes from within (pressures I put on myself)?*
2) *How much comes from external sources?*
3) *How do I react to outside pressure?*
4) *How many outside pressures have I taken in?*

What Is Your Idea of Happiness?

When they asked the great filmmaker Alfred Hitchcock at the end of his life for his idea of happiness, he answered "An empty horizon!"

One way of getting an idea of where you are at with stress is to ask:

1) *Can I be alone?*
2) *How do I feel when I am alone?*
3) *What thoughts occur?*
4) *What feelings occur?*

Golden Rule for the Week

By giving people the benefit of the doubt, we are really doing ourselves a favor. Imagining the best motives for others keeps *us* in a good frame of mind, which means a more relaxed and healthy state, especially for week four, antistress week!

"For centuries we've known that forgiving others is good for your spiritual health—now we know that it is good for your physical health as well. Forgiveness equals letting go of anger and pain—and that equals less stress!"
—Jane Clemen, Fight the Fat organizer

Want a good saying to help you when you clench your teeth and think of that X*?!#@!? Here's one written by the famous eighteenth-century French writer La Rochefoucauld: "We forgive to the extent that we love."

It's very easy to see the effects of holding on to anger. When the Iron Chancellor Bismarck wrote in his diary, "I was awake all night—*hating!*" he was describing a physical reaction to harboring dark thoughts about others. Dark, hostile personalities are taxing on your health: studies have shown anger and outbursts of temper to be a significant factor in heart attack and stroke patients. Given a choice between a hospital bed and *forgive and forget*, who wouldn't let bygones be bygones?

And while you're at it, forgive yourself, too! We've *all* made mistakes! Try it! You won't only *feel* lighter, you'll *become* lighter.

Food of the Week

Grapefruit. There's a reason why grapefruits have always been associated with weight loss—get hooked on this very special fruit and you've taken a giant step forward! Once you get in the grapefruit habit, its tart, juicy taste and its bulk can take the edge off your appetite before meals. This low-calorie food also prevents constipation and is a natural diuretic (gets rid of excess water). As if all this were not enough, it's a good source of vitamin C, calcium, and potassium. To get the juiciest grapefruits when shopping, lift up a dozen or so to get a sense of the weight. The heaviest has the most juice.

Vegetable Delight

Remember: you can eat all the vegetables you want, raw or cooked, spiced up or plain. Sometimes you just want to eat—and eat and eat. You want bulk. Vegetables can provide that along with taste if you dress them up. Even without getting fancy, you can add flavor by stir-frying them in a wok with Pam or with a teaspoon or two of olive oil or canola oil for a huge serving. Add some soy sauce, fresh pepper, and fresh lemon juice—*voila!* you can cook up a treat in no time. A subtler version of the stir-fry is below. There are literally hundreds of gourmet variations! Vinegar, poppy or sesame seeds, herbs, or Worcestershire sauce are other ways of making those greens *talk to you!*

One Fight the Fat member boiled her carrots with a touch of cinnamon and some fresh, grated ginger, and one half of a grated apple until there was very little water left in the pan. Then she put them in the refrigerator overnight—the result was naturally sweet and delicious. It was a simple discovery, but it kept her going during her daughter's birthday party where everyone else was eating cake and candy!

Share creative suggestions with your teammates. By putting your heads together, you get the combined results of your team's ingenuity and inspiration. There are wonderful fruit- and vegetable-based marinades that can turn vegetables into the hit of the meal—Apricot Garlic, Ginger Red Pepper, Tangerine Horseradish (it sounds strange but it's to die for!), and Wildberry Sage!

You can also get vegetable kabob mix at your supermarket, usually in the meat department. It's a package of already cut up mushrooms, onions, cabbage, and peppers, sometimes with skewers included. All you have to do is dip them in some soy or teriyaki sauce then throw them in the broiler or on the grill.

For people whose experience with veggies have been limited to cans of peas (how I was raised—peas are actually a starchy vegetable and higher in calories than others, by the way!), here's a good list of eat-all-you-want veggies to start you off: artichokes, asparagus, bamboo shoots, green and red peppers, lettuce, bean sprouts, beet greens, green beans, broccoli, cabbage, cauliflower, bok choy, celery, chicory, cabbage (sauerkraut), cucumbers, endives, mushrooms, kohlrabis, pimientos, radishes, spinach, summer squash, turnip greens, watercress, zucchini, carrots, and eggplant.

Okay! The following is a snack or meal idea that's based on vegetables and has gourmet taste. It is low-fat, low in calories, takes thirty minutes, and is inexpensive—who needs fast food?

Vegetable Stir-Fry
(To make this a main meal, spoon this stir-fry over soba or rice noodles. Makes four servings.)

1 tbsp. tamari or soy sauce
1 tbsp. rice wine vinegar (mild vinegar found in Asian markets)
1 tsp arrowroot mixed with 1 tbsp. vegetable broth
1 tsp olive oil
1 inch piece fresh ginger, cut into thin slices

1 clove garlic, minced

1 cup cauliflower

1 cup broccoli

½ cup vegetable broth *or* water

About ½ cup asparagus spears, chopped

½ cup thinly sliced zucchini

1 cup shiitake mushrooms

½ cup julienned red bell pepper

½ cup shelled edamame

¼ cup sliced scallions

1) Mix tamari, rice wine vinegar, and arrowroot until well blended. Set aside.

2) In nonstick wok or large skillet, heat oil over medium-high flame. Add ginger, garlic, cauliflower, and broccoli, and stir fry 3 minutes. Stir in ¼ cup broth.

3) Add asparagus, zucchini, mushrooms, bell pepper, and edamame. Stir-fry until vegetables are crisp, 2 minutes. Stir in remaining ¼ cup broth.

4) Stir in tamari mixture and cook 2 minutes. Stir in scallions. Remove ginger and season with salt and freshly ground pepper to taste. Serve hot.

(150 calories , 7 grams fat)

This really exciting stir-fry is by Louis Lanza, author of *Totally Dairy-Free Cooking*. He also has a really creative salad that shows you what you can do with vegetables when you put your mind to it.

Chopped Vegetable Salad

(The tempeh "bacon," avocado, and chickpeas in this recipe provide a protein powerhouse. Makes four servings.)

Vinaigrette

½ cup fresh carrot juice

½ cup extra-firm tofu, drained

1 tsp tamari or soy sauce

2 tsp tahini

1 tbsp. plus 1 tsp rice wine vinegar (mild vinegar found in Asian markets)

1 tsp dark sesame oil

2 tbsp. grated carrots

¼ cup diced tempeh "bacon" (2 strips)

4 cups chopped or julienned romaine lettuce

½ cup diced tomato

½ cup diced ripe avocado

½ cup canned chickpeas, rinsed and drained

½ cup seeded, diced cucumber

½ cup sliced Belgian endive

1) Make vinaigrette. In food processor or blender, combine carrot juice, tofu, tamari, tahini, vinegar, and oil, and process until blended. Transfer to bowl and stir in grated carrots. Cover and chill until ready to serve.

2) Lightly coat small, nonstick pan with cooking spray. Add diced "bacon" and cook, stirring often, until browned, 2 to 3 minutes. Transfer tempeh to plate.

3) In a bowl, combine lettuce, tomato, avocado, chickpeas, cucumber, endive, and ½ cup dressing. Toss to mix. Season with salt and freshly ground pepper to taste. Sprinkle with tempeh "bacon" and serve.

(154 calories, 8 grams fat)

Okay! These recipes should help convince you that vegetables can become a *main attraction,* the staple of your menu. It's all about investing a little time and effort in your meal planning—and this is one investment you can't go wrong with. The payoff is a healthier you!

Self-empowerment Exercise for the Week

Building bridges to the past. "The past is always with us," says Dr. Brenda Shoshanna, author of *Zen Miracles*. "Sometimes it acts as a positive force in our lives, sometimes as a negative one. Examine something painful in your life and think about what you have learned from it. We can and must learn something from every experience that we have undergone!"

Some strength, some wisdom, some insight is to be found in all suffering. Just knowing that you can survive a tragedy is empowering—focus on what good can come out of the painful experience you have had.

When you find yourself having overwhelming urges to eat, take that first step away from compulsive eating by pausing. Do not give in to the urge right away. I will eat in ten minutes, or a half-hour—tell yourself and mean it!

But use the time you have bought to think of what is behind the urge. If past issues are behind the craving, work with them! See what good came out of your experiences instead of remaining locked into an "I didn't want this to happen" mode.

Even if this is difficult at first, repeated practice will make it an easier and more natural process. Another advantage is that often food urges run their course. They surge and then slowly fade. If you can wait them out while you reach for your journal instead of for that candy bar, you are building emotional muscle. Keep making the *waiting time* longer. Keep focusing on the emotional part of the hunger.

Instead of eating to forget, face what you are trying to forget, remember everything, and learn.

Stress Antidote for the Week

Take a bath. In the nineteenth century, they used warm water to soothe lunatics. In the twentieth century, everyone qualifies for this treatment! Spas understand the value of water therapy, offering their guests such specialties as mineral baths, aroma-therapeutic soaks, private whirlpools, and elaborate five-stage Roman baths. The Russian baths in New York City have alternating pools of steaming hot and cold water and offer a birch-wood cleansing in addition to massage. But you can get started with a simple but effective "spa" of your own. Make the following a habit (two or three times a week), and by the end of a month you will see a huge difference in the way you feel. What? Who has time for this? You do. Me? The new you!

After warning your family, make up a strong sign. It should send this message:

Working toward the new me!
I will not take phone calls!
If you care about my health,
if you care about me,
do not disturb please!
I am doing this for my health and sanity!
Respect my wishes!
Thank you!

Make sure that the kids get the message: they will lose big time if they interrupt you for anything except a medical emergency! After a while, family members will automatically accept the change. "Mom's taking her bath" or "Dad's chilling out" will become an accepted part of the new routine that you have made. But you have to stand up for yourself and stick to your guns.

The bathroom will be your inner sanctum for the half-hour or the hour you have put aside.

Research has shown that smell and taste exert a strong influence over our moods. The Smell & Taste Treatment & Research Foundation in Chicago has lauded the scent of green apples as an antidepressant, and lavender and chamomile have been found to be great for stress relief as well. You can buy a wide variety of stress-relieving scented candles to give a soft glow to the darkened bathroom. Pour the lavender and chamomile oils into the hot water.

Turn on the soothing music—choose it with care. Something soft, without words, perhaps something exotic. It might be that you just want a tape with the sound of the ocean, which has a very basic, very comforting message. As you lie in the water, you can adjust your breathing to the rhythm of the ocean. Try to concentrate on your breaths and on the sounds. If other thoughts occur, let them go and gently refocus on the waves.

If you've chosen music to listen to, do the same thing, concentrating on the music, on the candles, on the scents and sensation of the water. Keep your attention focused on the here and now.

This is a crucial part of the treatment: let go of stressful thought, worry, and the cares of the day. Dr. Benson, associate professor of medicine at Harvard Medical School and author of *The Relaxation Response* and *Beyond The Relaxation Response,* explains that "The relaxation response is a bodily capacity that's the exact opposite of the stress response." Stress causes the heart rate to rise, the metabolism to increase, and the body to release adrenaline. The muscles tense. Anger and hostility take over. When you go into a deeply relaxed state, the opposite of all these physical processes occurs. (Although the bath is an ideal setting, Dr. Benson's books can guide you to working out all kinds of variations on this theme, places and environments that can help you achieve this supremely calm state.)

The smells, sounds, and sensations of your bath are aids that you must allow to work on you by becoming passive. Image: you are a leaf floating in the pond. That is all you have to do. Lie there and float! Or block out all thoughts by repeating a single word (a mantra) like "love" or "peace." These simple techniques can bring about health-enhancing physiological changes—as the yoga practitioners and meditation gurus have known for a long time. If someone could sell you these in a bottle for one hundred dollars a pill and no side effects, you'd buy them! Here, all you need is to be willing to try out some new techniques and repeat the experiment over a period of time. And if you are, you will see the difference yourself.

Allow yourself this complete relaxation experience, and emerge from the water a "new you."

Chapter Five: Who *Is* That?

"I am not one of those people who claims she loves to exercise.
I simply love all that it does for me."
—Oprah Winfrey

"If I knew I was going to live this long, I'd have taken better care of myself."
—Adolph Zukor, legendary film producer, after reaching his one hundredth birthday

If you think exercise is a pain, try having a heart attack.
—Ad on a gym bag

Statistic: subjects enrolled in a hospital-based program at St. Francis Medical Center in Illinois were *twice as likely* to keep to their walking regimen for a year if they walked together with a partner.

Gyms are places where the fit go to get fitter—right? Wrong. Excuse me, Miss Body Beautiful, but is this machine taken? Make room for me! Fight the Fat flash. *You don't have to be an Olympic gold medal winner to get on a treadmill!* To use the words of the *Millennium Grannies* team captain, "Move whatever you can!" Word on the Fight the Fat block is that that's the key for all of us, whatever our age. A lot of what is called aging is just not using your body—you lose flexibility, you lose strength, you lose stamina. But you can get it back if you just start *moving! That* can be you in the gym mirror, dancing to the music!

Shocking Statistics
- Recommended exercise time for your health: thirty minutes a day! Just thirty minutes!
- Studies report that only 15 percent of Americans are getting it!

- Forty percent get *none at all!*
- Among high school students (your most active years), the number of active teenagers has dropped from 42 percent to 29 percent!

Fight the Fat organizer Dianna Kirkwood is unfazed by such statistics. "Here in Dyersville, we've turned those numbers around! Everybody is walking, marching, running, stretching. If you don't believe me, just go outside around five P.M. and see how many *older* people you'll see on bikes or power walking up a storm!

"That is because when you're on a team or have a weight buddy (who might have been your old eating buddy!) you can have *fun* exercising. And we need fun in our lives—we need to play, to bring out the inner child, to get in touch with the warmth and energy we used to have before all the so-called serious stuff got to us!"

In the beginning, of course, no one thinks of exercise this way. You haven't moved forever, exercise is difficult and makes you uncomfortable, and we all tend to take the path of least resistance. Most of the members I talked to hadn't really envisioned themselves in a gym when they joined. But they saw *Fight the Fat!* signs everywhere, and took the plunge with their eyes closed or half-closed. Once they joined, their teams scheduled exercise sessions and they just "kind of got swept along in the momentum of the thing" as Bonnie says, a young mother from New Vienna.

"There's a team called *No Excuses,*" she recalls, "and that's how I felt when I sat down with other women who were just as busy as I was but who seemed to have no qualms about spending all this time getting healthy. I kept thinking, *What have I gotten myself into?* And that wasn't only at the first meeting. It took about two months until I was really committed to exercising the way they were and feeling, *Yes—I can do this. I can keep it up.*"

What kept Bonnie going those two months? Part of it was the team (once she got to know them better, teammates told her that they had had just as many doubts as she had). The other part was her husband: "He told me I was wasting my money by joining and I wanted to prove him wrong.

He got my goat by just assuming I'd drop out. That made me have an *I'll show him* attitude. Another factor was a neighbor down the block and I think I couldn't have faced her either every day if I'd quit. I don't want to go into details, but she'd made some pretty snide remarks to me about my weight. But now I don't care what she or anyone else thinks—I exercise for myself. I've really gotten into it."

Teams organized many events for themselves, including cardio-exercise classes (like spin classes), volley ball matches, races, and Sunday hikes together with team *and* family members (followed by picnics with smart choices from Fight the Fat menus). There were also basketball games and row boating events on the Mississippi. This kind of variety gave a real boost to everyone's determination to keep active. The games weren't *fight to the finish.* There was a lot of laughter on both sides of the volleyball court. But there was also a lot of pride. People were regaining the use of their bodies and felt good about it.

Another reason for the enthusiasm was the steady progress brought about by the exercise classes. The class I attended in Dyersville was given by a wonderful instructor, Sue Engelbrecht, who had made the class special with a mixture of humor, inspirational quotes, music, and exercises that everyone could participate in no matter what their fitness level.

As if she was putting together a healthy recipe, Sue threw in some meditation between the strenuous workouts: a few thoughts for her teammates to take away with them. And I can tell you from this experience that when you are resting between sets, recovering and breathing deeply, everything you hear during that time has an additional impact. During those pauses, you can really hear the truth of what she is saying—all that physical activity has opened you up and made you forget your normal concerns and worries and even your self-consciousness. It was a great experience.

Then there were the walkathons each week after the large Fight the Fat meetings. Everybody was revved up and put more into the power walk. I didn't see one person drop out. The captain of the Dyersville ten-member team *Getting Fit* said, "With the energy from the meeting still in the air, these walkathons were a great way to start off our new week." It's no mystery why her team lost over two hundred pounds together during the campaign.

This scene becomes all the more impressive when you consider that most of these people have already put in a long day and have other responsibilities and chores at night as well. Take Sara, a nurse and young mother who joined another ten-member Dyersville team called *The Resolutions* together with her mother, who also needed to lose some weight, "I do medical, surgical, nursery, and labor delivery at Mercy Medical Center," she told me during her lunch break. "At times it gets really stressful.

"I guess that's why it took me a whole year until I joined Fight the Fat —the first time I just sat it out and watched—and listened. I thought I didn't have the time. And then the second year I had so much weight to lose that I almost passed it up again. I thought, *What's the use?* But I did join at the last minute and I took off twenty-three pounds during those ten weeks and then twenty pounds after that—that was last year.

"But still I was very slow getting into exercise. Somewhere in the middle of the campaign, though, I caught on—*exercise is something I do for myself,*" she said with emphasis.

"My husband is very supportive," she went on. "He's very athletic himself. It's hard to fit in exercise with a husband and three kids; and he once offered to watch them while I ran and I never let him off the hook after that! Sometimes my mom helps out with the kids, too. But even if I have to hire a baby-sitter to be able to exercise, I will. I've come to learn that I need it for my mood as much as I do physically. It's my time for myself. This year I'm going to do walking, aerobics, and bike riding. I'm looking forward to it now. I love it."

Members who met with their group just once a week to exercise found that that "push" kept them going on their own during the rest of the week. They wanted to be able to keep up with their team members the next time they met.

A member of the seniors team, the *Millennium Grannies,* combats the *I don't feel like doing it today* syndrome by combining *realism* and *optimism* and coming up with a thought that's helpful to people of all ages. "When people get old, they don't think they need exercise. But exercise is even more important when you are in the sunset of life. Some older people keep saying, *I can't, I can't*—but the truth is *they can.* That's my message to other seniors. Get started doing *something,* even if it's only wriggling your fingers and toes. Afterwards, you'll be surprised how much more you are gradually able to do."

In addition to all the benefits mentioned so far, exercise also depresses your appetite and elevates your mood, releasing natural substances called endorphins in the brain. The old joke used to be *When I feel like exercising, I lie down until the feeling passes.* But that's an old joke—and the joke was on us! Now, with a grin on our faces from those endorphins released by a brisk, twenty-minute walk, we can truly say *When I feel like eating, I exercise until the urge goes away!*

Fight the Fat Advice

The following is advice gleaned from Fight the Fat speakers, Fight the Fat members, and Fight the Fat founders. Pay attention! If you know what you're doing, then you'll do it right!

Hydration

First of all, drink! Drink! Drink! Never dehydrate when you're working out. Keep a bottle of water nearby! This is essential.

Next, an ounce of prevention—when exercising, wear cotton-crotch or all-cotton underwear. Cotton absorbs moisture better. Don't lounge around in tight pants and synthetic tights. When you finish exercising, take them off. To fight bacteria, always change out of sweaty gym clothes or wet bathing suits as soon as possible.

Heart Rate

Is your heart rate too high or too low when you work out? The American College of Sports Medicine guideline for cardiovascular training is work within 60 to 80 percent of your maximum heart rate when you exercise. *How do I know what this is?*

> Method #1: Using your first two fingers (not your thumb), press to the point where you can feel your pulse (either in your wrist or neck). Count the number of pulses you feel in ten seconds. What you want is about twenty-four pulses in ten seconds, which equals one hundred and forty-four per minute, approximately 70 percent of your capacity.

> Method #2: The target heart rate zone for weight loss is 65 to 80 percent of your maximum heart rate. You can estimate your maximum heart rate by subtracting your age from 220.

Or, let the machine do it for you! Use a heart monitor. The monitor makes sure you're in touch with your body's capability. It gives you feedback on the spot. You can chart your progress and compete with yourself in a sensible way. And that will keep you going!

Either way, staying within your comfort zone prevents you from feeling like a wet noodle afterwards—sore and exhausted. And we're talking not quitting here!

The opposite can also be true: sometimes you're taking it too easy. Monitoring your heart will tell you that you can increase your speed somewhat or take a hill or an incline! The idea is to keep challenging yourself, and to keep winning—by losing!

The American Heart Association, the Surgeon General's Office, and countless health organizations have recommended strength training *in addition to* aerobics. Here are a few tips for those ready to begin weight training.

Weight Training: Improving Muscle Strength and Endurance

When you increase your lean body weight (that is, your muscle mass) you speed up your body's metabolism, which in turn increases the number of calories you burn up! By improving your lean-to-fat-weight ratio, and combining regular aerobic exercise (walking, biking, stepping) and weight training (dumbbells, bungee cords, weight lifting machines), your body will burn more calories, *both during exercise and at rest.*

Here are some basic guidelines for beginning a weight training program. When beginning, the main focus on the muscle is increasing muscle endurance. Here you want to start with lighter weights, or resistance, and perform a higher number of repetitions and sets. This is also appropriate for those people interested in improving muscle tone.

Example. Use one or two plates, or light weights that can be lifted up to fifteen times. Rest for thirty seconds to one minute. Then try to lift the weight fifteen times again; rest again and repeat. It should get more challenging during the second and third sets. In fact, you may not be able to reach fifteen repetitions on the second or third set. If you are able to reach fifteen just as easily on the first, second, and third sets, you could probably increase the weight slightly.

For increasing muscle strength, and for more definition, the idea is to increase the resistance and lower the number of repetitions and sets. This approach is appropriate for the intermediate to experienced weight lifter, and even then should be introduced modestly.

Example: one or two more weighted plates than usual to start out with. This can be increased depending on the individual, their goals, and health status. Lift the weight for up to ten to twelve times; rest for thirty seconds to one minute, and then repeat for a second set only. Again, you may not be able to reach the same number of repetitions on the second set. When you can reach the same number of repetitions consistently, for two weeks or so, you may either increase the weight slightly, or keep the weight the same to maintain the muscle tone and strength you've achieved.

Remember, these are general guidelines. Begin slowly and cautiously. Muscle soreness is common for the first week or so after beginning a weight lifting program. Muscle pain or persistent soreness may be a sign of injury. Investigate before continuing the weight training program.

Weight training tips:
• Lift the weight slowly.
• Always *exhale* on the lift, and *inhale* on the decline.
• Never hold your breath.

The weight stack should not come in contact with the rest of the stack inbetween repetitions. The bungee cord should not become slack between pulls. (This causes muscle relaxation between lifts, slows improvement, and may increase the risk of muscle injury.)

Figuring the Angles: Activity and Weight Loss

There are many charts giving the calorie counts for exercises ranging from walking to fencing! On the next page, we include a few examples so that you can get a sense of what you are actually burning off when you take to the treadmill.

(To make these numbers more impressive, just add a zero. Multiply them by ten minutes. For example, if you stay on that bike for ten minutes, those nine and a half calories turn into ninety-five. Make that a half-hour and you've worked off almost three hundred calories on your ride!)

An Amazing Fact

Bobbi Schell, Supervisor of Rehabilitation Outreach Services at Mercy, discussed muscle versus fat. "Because you are exercising you will be gaining muscle tissue. Muscles are denser, heavier, [and] weigh more than fat tissue, and you may be disappointed that your weight loss is not as fast as you wanted it to be in the beginning, or even that you gained a pound or two. But over time those pounds will come off.

"That's the bad news about muscles. The good news is that a muscular body burns calories at a higher rate. While you're sleeping, [or] while you're reading on a lounge chair, those muscles are working for you and telling your body, *Burn those calories faster!* Along with looking good, muscles speed up your metabolism. For every pound of muscle added to your

Activity	Calories Burned Per Minute	Activity	Calories Burned Per Minute
Aerobics	7.1	Running at 5 Miles Per Hour	9.5
Basketball	9.5	Running, Cross Country	10.7
Biking—Moderate	9.5	Running in Place	9.5
Biking—Leisurely	7.1	Sex—Moderate Sex	1.5
Boating	2.9	Sex—Vigorous Sex	1.7
Bowling	3.5	Shopping	2.7
Canoeing	4.7	Showering	4.7
Cooking	3	Sitting	1.2
Dancing	5.3	Skiing	8.3
Driving	2.3	Sleeping	1
Fishing	4.7	Soccer	8.5
Football	9.5	Stairmaster	7.1
Frisbee	3.5	Standing	1.4
Gardening	6	Stationary Bike	7.1
Golf	5.3	Studying at Desk	2.1
Hiking	7.1	Swimming	9.5
Horseback Riding	4.7	Talking on Phone	1.1
Housekeeping	2.9	Tennis	8.2
Office Work	1.7	Volleyball	3.5
Playing Piano	2.9	Walking—	
Playing Guitar	3.5	Less Than 2 Miles Per Hour	2.3
Playing with Kids	5	Walking—	
Racquet Ball	11.9	4.5 Miles Per Hour	5.3
Reading	1.1	Watching Television	1.1
Rock Climbing	13.1	Weight lifting	3.5
Rowing	6	Writing	1.1
Running up Stairs	18	Yoga	4.7

Source: American Heart Association and John Hopkins University

body, you'll burn at least thirty-five more calories per day. Three pounds of muscle will burn enough calories in a month to lose a pound of fat! You are burning extra calories even when you rest in order to support the heavier muscle tissue!

"This is one way that you can really melt off those pounds in your sleep! *Use strength training for weight loss success!*"

Walking—for the Mind and the Body
Power Walking

Power walking requires you to pick up the pace and challenge yourself to increase your walking speed. If you are conversing as you walk, you aren't at a challenging level. Your arms swing forward with elbows bent at ninety-degree angles, propelling your body forward. Your back is upright and your stomach is tucked in. You can do this for the entire walk, but if you are a beginner it may work better to power walk in intervals, which requires you to pick up the pace to a power walk for thirty seconds at a time. Later, you can increase the power-walk interval up to three to four minutes with a two-to-three-minute slow down between each power walk.

Walking Tips

Fight the Fat organizer Dianna Kirkwood: "There is a scene from *Good Morning, Vietnam* where Robin Williams plays the part of a DJ pretending to be a fashion consultant. The make-believe consultant doesn't get the point of camouflage. He reasons that the troops are in battle and suggests that the wardrobe should clash! I was thinking of that as I drove to work the other day. I see walkers every morning. Some I see a block off with their [reflective] clothes. Others you would think were on a reconnaissance mission. When you walk, please follow Robin's advice and be highly visible. And not just when it's dark: dawn and dusk have their own visibility problems."

Walking is a great stress reliever and a good cardiovascular workout (at a brisk pace for an uninterrupted twenty minutes). But besides these benefits, walking is often the best way to solve problems and lift your mood. Such great minds and spirits as Albert Einstein, Charles Dickens, Thomas Jefferson, and Harry Truman took daily brisk walks to think out their problems (you're in good company!). You may be more worried about paying the bills than the speed of light, but after a walk the cleared, relaxed mind can think of alternatives you would have overlooked in your harried, stressed-out state.

When is the best time to walk? Anytime. If you walk after a meal, take it slow to help digestion (actually, this is a particularly good time to walk since after a meal you are giving your body the message: don't store these calories as fat! You raise the metabolic rate and begin to burn off the food you've taken in right away). If the weather is too hot, wait until the sun goes down.

The weekends are great for hikes. More and more events like the state games feature walks along with runs and other such events. If you wish to pack in some additional activity when walking, increase your speed or do the stairs. Stairs increase the effort by 400 percent.

But don't worry about stairs at first. The main thing is to make a beginning, and walking is a terrific way since it requires no equipment, no gyms, nothing special. You're on your way to get something from a neighbor a few blocks away. You are about to get into your car—are you kidding? You know what you have to do!

Your Workbook

Exercises, Questions, Tips, & Points to Ponder for Week 5 of Fight the Fat

The Bulletin Board

"I write when I'm inspired—but I make sure that
I'm inspired at nine o' clock every morning."
—Peter De Vries, novelist

"Life is like a ten-speed bike. We all have gears we never use."
—Charles Schultz

"We can't take any credit for our talents. It's how we use them that counts."
—Madeleine L'Engle

The following gems are from Dyersville Fight the Fat Notices for the spring 2000 campaign.

"People tend to think on a grand scale or plan super initiatives. This is all well and good, but the 'devil is in the details.' Having titanic plans and shooting for super health is a great goal. But you need to focus on the process, the countless small steps to your goal."

"Lance Armstrong is a world-class cyclist who [recovered] from cancer. His attitude was that there were two kinds of days—good days and great days. This is an observation common among those who have an increased appreciation for life. May you enjoy that view without any bad health. Have a month filled with good and great days."

Given any thought to Ping-Pong lately? In the early 1900s, the game experienced a short but intense popularity boom. The mini-craze led to some good and bad outcomes. The bad was evident in an outbreak of wrist tendonitis. On the other hand, women's fashions changed to allow looser clothing to facilitate the movement necessary for a good game of Ping-Pong. Ping-Pong anyone?

The late comedian Jack Benny was known as a skinflint. He had a routine where he was held up and told *Your money or your life!* Jack stood there without answering until finally the bandit shouted, *Well?*

Shush! Jack shouted back at him *I'm thinking! I'm thinking!"*

We laugh at Jack's dilemma—of course the sight of someone choosing money over his life is absurd. But the same is true about all those extra pounds you're carrying around. The thief is trying to rob you of your health and long life. The thief is saying to you, *Your ice cream, your potato chips, your Ding Dongs, or your life!* Put that way, it sounds just as absurd, doesn't it? — Dianna Kirkwood, Fight the Fat organizer, with an interesting slant on the weight issue

Your Journal

Marion Bilich, author of *Weight Loss from the Inside Out,* says, "Sometimes a man or a woman will not be able to lose weight or get over an eating problem completely because the problem itself is serving a function in his or her life." How many times do we blame everything on our weight! I'll go out and socialize more—*when I am thin.* I can't exercise (or travel, go out to singles parties, etc.) now—but I'll start when I'm thin. Weight can be a way we have of endlessly putting off activities that make us anxious or uncomfortable. Or, we may focus on food as a way of not considering other problems in our life.

Consider these issues in your journal. Ask yourself these questions:

1) *How will my life be different when I am fit?*
2) *What thoughts/images immediately come to mind?*
3) *How do they make me feel?*

Do some soul-searching this week! It may be painful—but not as painful as eating yourself into oblivion!

Healthy Habit for the Week

Write down everything you eat! This is a hard one at first, but it pays big dividends. *It's such a pain! Why do I have to do this?* is a frequent response. The answer is *You don't have to, but it really helps.* Studies in other areas of compulsive behavior (such as compulsive spending) demonstrate that this is a key to gaining control over addictive behavior. (Compulsive spenders keep track of every penny they spend during a day.)

Writing makes you aware of what you're doing—really aware, step-by-step. Half the time you put food in your mouth without even thinking about it. It's as if you never had it!

But once you *write down* how many spoonfuls of that ice cream you've had, you're introducing a measure of control. Pretend that you had a partner in a business who was given to "borrowing" a little petty cash from the register every now and then. Wouldn't you want her to write it down so that you knew exactly how much? The same idea applies here. When at the end of the day you look up calorie values, you can see just how much "petty cash" you're borrowing—sometimes that "petty cash" is enough to buy a Rolls Royce!

Writing things down keeps you honest! One member uses a beautiful pocket-sized diary with inspiring sayings across the top of each page and photos of flowers! She even scents the book with a drop or two of perfume. But even if you end up scribbling down notes to yourself on the cardboard from your panty hose it's good enough. "Writing brings control!" says Fight the Fat organizer Jane Clemen.

Reward for the Week

A special *treat*ment—guilt-free pleasure. *On occasion,* it is a good thing to reward yourself with a *portion* of the sinfully rich food you used to eat all the time! (Note the emphases in this sentence: *on occasion* and *a portion.* The *occasion* is your reward week. And *a portion* can be found in any good nutritional book. See the bibliography for several of them).

There are two reasons for this. The first is that by eating this food in a controlled way, you are preventing these foods from developing a "mystique"—from having a power over you. Things that are forbidden have a way of becoming more wonderful by the day. As King Solomon said, "Stolen waters are sweeter." You remember that special cake or cookie as being even better and more delicious than they really were.

So, take the mystery out of them—but eat them in controlled circumstances. The second reason for this experiment/exercise/reward: *willpower is like a muscle! The more you use it, the stronger it becomes!*

Think about it! When you eat four ounces of the rich ice cream you used to have by the quart, you are sending yourself a message. *Now I am in control!* You are building self-respect. And you are enjoying the ice cream, too, by the way!

If you can buy just so much and no more of a treat, for example, two or three of those delicious cookies you used to eat by the pound, then buy just that number. Ignore the voice telling you, "Well isn't it ridiculous to go all the way to the bakery for three cookies? I'll just pick up a pound for my neighbor, my husband, or the elderly lady down the block." Forget those missions of mercy. You'll end up eating the whole pound yourself.

If you feel you have to explain at the bakery why you're only buying two or three, say that you're on a diet—it's no big shame! Twenty-five percent of Americans are overweight! If the food cannot be bought in a single-portion size, then try *throwing out or giving away what you are not going to eat before you take a taste.*

Of course, *Never throw away food!* is the mantra we were raised on. And our parents were right; waste is a bad thing. But, in our affluent society there is often a huge surplus of leftovers and we end up becoming human disposal machines! You are helping no one by consuming whatever is left over! And think of this treat as part of a *treatment*, a process of turning those old destructive pleasures into part of your new, healthy lifestyle.

If you plan on regularly giving yourself this kind of reward (say, once a week), then you have to analyze the calorie content of your treat and work it into the mathematics of your weight loss plan (see chapter 7 for this). But if it's a one-time deal, forget it! No one ever got fat from *one* piece of cake or *one* four-ounce serving of ice cream.

Enjoy! Remember, the best ingredient in your treat: it is guilt-free!

Team Activity for the Week

Portion control! "We tend to eat what's put in front of us, and portions in this country are huge!" says Dr. Barbara Rolls, professor of nutrition at Penn State and author of *Volumetrics.*

Teams in Dyersville worked on portion control together in a fun way: they used guessing games. Each member had to bring in five or six foods that people commonly grab for a snack—a bagel, a bag of fries or popcorn, a muffin, etc. Then, after "eyeballing" it, the other members "voted"—figuring out weight, calories, grams of fat, and, *hardest of all*, what should be considered a portion for one person.

Take a look at some examples of "food inflation" in recent years. French fries have gone from two ounces to four or more. Bagels have gone from two to seven ounces. Muffins have gone from two ounces to six to eight ounces. Soda has gone from six and a half ounces to twelve to twenty ounces. A small bag of chips has gone from one ounce to four ounces!

Golden Rule for the Week

Eat a hearty, healthy breakfast! Don't think of it as a meal. Think of it as a *preventive measure!* Studies show that people who skip breakfast tend to eat out of control later on in the day! Breakfast is such an important meal because it is just that—the breaking of a fast. A large breakfast helps you get into high gear by speeding up the metabolism. After hours of working on low gear during sleep, you are giving your body the right signal—speed up! This allows you to burn more calories as you prepare for your well-balanced day.

Complaint: "I'm just not hungry in the morning!" Answer: "It doesn't matter. Skip breakfast and you run a higher chance of getting into trouble later on."

Breakfast is a crucial part of that other healthy habit you've gotten into—eating small, frequent meals or healthy snacks spaced every few hours to keep the blood sugar at a good level. That higher level of blood sugar gives you energy and helps put you in a good mood. How many arguments can be traced to low blood sugar level stemming from deprivation!

Skipping meals contributes to obesity just as much as overeating!

A Breakfast Suggestion

Forget the bacon and eggs—you don't need all that fat. Think grains. They're high in fiber (fiber makes you feel full, helps digestion, and is a way of preventing colon cancer) and they're also high in B vitamins. Oat bran is especially good since it has the added advantage of controlling cholesterol. If you're pressed for time in the morning, *take the time* to make a satisfying and nutritious breakfast the night before and heat it up in the morning. Imagine starting the day with the following example of a healthy breakfast—believe me, you won't be tempted by the sugar doughnuts brought around at the office and you are less likely to be affected by mid-morning slump.

Fruit & Kashi Eye Opener!

Kashi—*don't confuse it with its healthy cousin, kasha.* Kashi is a multigrain mixture you can find at natural food stores. This recipe will get you off to a good start in the morning:

1 cup cooked Kashi pilaf cereal
1 apple, minced (or: 1 cup of strawberries, 1 banana, 1 pear, etc.)
1 tsp lemon juice
1 tsp vanilla or almond extract
Cinnamon or ginger to taste

Mix and bake at 400° for about one-half hour.

2 servings are approximately 175 calories.

Banana Smoothie

1 frozen banana (never throw 'em out when they get ripe: freeze 'em).

½ cup nonfat yogurt

½ cup fresh orange juice

¼ cup blueberries or strawberries

Blend until smooth.

Food of the Week

Fish. There's nothing fishy about fish! For the protein it provides, it's amazingly low in calories. It averages about one hundred calories per ounce (shellfish is about eighty calories, abalone is at the low end of the scale with sixty-seven calories per ounce, herring is at the top with 177 calories per ounce, and water-packed tuna comes in at about 115 calories per ounce). When you're shopping for your dinner, look for firm flesh, tight scales, red gills, clear eyes, and a fresh smell.

The benefits are enormous: a major source of protein, fish has far less saturated fat than meat, and eaten several times a week, it has been connected to a lower risk of heart attack, stroke, and breast cancer. The oils in fish thin the blood, reduce blood pressure, and lower cholesterol. Fish lovers have higher levels of HDL (that's the "good" cholesterol that is protective). Finally, fish is thought to be a tumor inhibitor and an anti-inflammatory (research is still studying these and other benefits).

For a really healthy meal, why not use calcium-rich kale as a wrap when steaming fillet of fish (see Workbook for Week Three)?

Just to start you thinking *fish,* here are a few fish recipes that are mouth-watering.

Fish Kabob

With dishes like this, you don't miss meat. I had this in a Dyersville restaurant, and it was so good I got the recipe on the spot!

½ cup lemon juice

1 tbsp. oil

Ginger to taste

1 tbsp. parsley

1 pound fresh filets (fish of your choice)

About 1 pound mushrooms

1 red pepper, diced

1 onion, diced

1 large cauliflower

1) Cut fish into cubes and marinate in lemon juice, oil, and ginger for about two hours.
2) Drain and skewer the fish along with the mushrooms, peppers, onions, and cauliflower.
3) Dip the kabobs in marinade and broil three to ten minutes (watch out, don't let it burn!).
4) Dip again in marinade and broil about ten minutes more.

This recipe makes two servings.

Oriental Salmon: *Best-Loved Fish Meal* in a Fight the Fat survey!

Fillet of fresh salmon, 8 ounces

⅓ cup rice wine vinegar

¼ cup orange marmalade

2 tbsp. teriyaki sauce

1 tbsp. grated, fresh ginger root

2 tsp sesame oil

6-ounce package of wild rice, cooked without salt. (You can get a great package of rice at Trader Joe's called Rice Trilogy—it's made up of California brown basmati rice, California long grain branch, and

California wild rice.)
¾ cup fresh snow pea pods
½ cup sliced green onions
½ cup chopped sweet red bell pepper
Bibb lettuce leaves

1) Place salmon in an eight-inch square dish and set aside.
2) Combine vinegar, marmalade, teriyaki sauce, and grated ginger root in a jar.
3) Cover tightly and shake well.
4) Pour half of the mixture over the salmon.
5) Turn.
6) Set aside leftover mixture.
7) Drain salmon, discard marinade.
8) Place salmon on a rack in broiler pan.
9) Broil five minutes on each side.

Ali K.'s Unscientific Tartar Sauce

(This is an all-time winner! Surveyed, it's off the charts!) Use as a dip for fish or as a base for salad dressing.
2 fresh, squeezed lemons
2 tsp chopped, fresh garlic
Fresh dill, no stems
2 finely chopped dill pickles
Parsley
2 capfuls of vinegar
Light mayonnaise—amount depends on desired consistency
Salt and pepper to taste

Combine all of the ingredients in a bowl. Whisk together and pop in the freezer for twenty minutes to a half-hour (until it gels).

Self-empowerment Exercise for the Week

Connect with a higher power. The twelve-step programs understand the significance of getting out of the "me" syndrome—being obsessed with "self" is a sure formula for misery. That's why these programs work. It doesn't matter what your beliefs are. What matters is that you feel connected with a force larger than yourself. For some it is the wonder of nature, for others the beauty of art—even the atheist Karl Marx "believed" in the value of social justice and its inevitable triumph! As Oscar Wilde put it, "A cynic is a person who knows the price of everything—and the value of nothing." When you get in touch with your values, you are getting in touch with a sustaining, motivating, strengthening force. Too many of us rush through our days without tapping in!

Dr. Frederic Flach, M.D., author of *Resilience: Discovering a New Strength at Times Of Stress*, found that survivors, people who overcome all kinds of adversity, have in common a deep sense of meaning and purpose in their lives. This can come from their belief in God, or it can come from a personal philosophy or system of values that teach them that every human being is unique and precious regardless of what he or she achieves or fails to achieve. In other words, you are one of a kind! When they made you they broke the mold! The world is a better place because you are in it!

To go with your outer makeover from last week, work on an "inner makeover" this week. Modern life makes so many demands on us and is so rushed that most people don't stop to think about the *why*—they're too busy with the *how*.

Get together with your teammates to discuss an inspirational book that you have chosen together. It can be fiction or nonfiction, a novel, a play, a biography, a first person narrative of adversity overcome, or a fascinating glimpse into a life such as Helen Keller's or Anne Frank's. As Dr. Andrew Weil observes after a lifetime of seeing patients, "People who experience themselves as part of and supported by something larger than themselves are less fearful and more healthy than people who view the world through the bars of an ego cage, seeing the world as separate from them, disconnected."

Stress Antidote for the Week

"The real voyage of discovery consists not in just seeing
new landscapes, but in having new eyes."
—Marcel Proust

Try either body-style gardening (calorie burning), or soul-style gardening (spirit nourishing)! That's right, there are two kinds—and both get an *A-Plus* as stress reducers.

Body-style gardening is heavy-duty stuff that is not for everybody. But you can start off slow, scatter a few hardy seeds in the spring (like morning glory or marigold), plant a few sturdy vines (like clematis or wisteria), and you've added a whole new dimension to your life. Just watching something you've planted grow or burst into blossom is rewarding.

Many Fight the Fat members report that once you get in the swing of it, you're surprised by how gratifying and pleasurable it is. As Eileen of Dyersville told me during a Fight the Fat rally, "Before I started gardening, I was so tired at the end of the day! If my kids wanted something, if my husband wanted something, everyone got the same answer—I'd done enough. But after getting into gardening, I *love* to go out to the flower beds when I come home. I lose myself in the shrubs. When I am in my garden, [this] feeling comes over me. *It doesn't get any better.* It really calms me down. You want something from me. The time to ask is after I've been gardening!"

And Eileen is talking serious movement here. All the blood, sweat, and tears involved in gardening—the hoeing, piling compost, weeding, etc.— burn more calories than a step aerobics class according to the *Green Gym* in England (an organization that encourages people to lose weight while improving the environment).

What a payoff: beautiful colors and scents, better body tone, burned-off fat, and stress reduction (a better mental outlook). That's why gardening is the No. 1 hobby in this country.

There are few satisfactions like watering and pruning and getting into a deeper relationship with the earth. Even seeing a houseplant thrive under your hands can be a source of joy. Gardening, at any level, draws you out and teaches you patience. Even during the winter, your garden can take your mind off worries. The catalogs to order from are a feast for the eyes—there are endless varieties of almost every garden flower and shrub. The planning and the anticipation are half the fun.

Gardening clubs are very popular since members swap tips and suggestions. Ask your fellow teammates whether there are any gardeners among them? Would the team care to include a gardening event during the summer or a visit to a botanical garden? Flowers soothe, stimulate, and inspire. Shift the focus from sweets to scents.

Margaret of Dubuque combined her gardening with a passion for photography and started a photo album of her garden and of gardens that she admired. She had close-ups of flowers that were works of art— a spectacular photo of a tulip, or a shot of a rose bush just about to burst into bloom decorated the rooms of her house. It brought her, and me, joy to look at them.

She said, "I began during my first Fight the Fat. Usually I'd ask my son to rake the leaves, but that year I decided to do it myself for the exercise. I found [that] I liked being outdoors (I had and still have an unused treadmill sitting in my basement). I'm the kind of person who just can't stand going into a gym. But I noticed that the raking made me feel invigorated. So, I put in some late autumn mums, and that was the beginning of it all. My garden has given me so much happiness that I am a much different person from the old me."

A final suggestion is an *herb garden:* add fresh sprigs of basil, oregano, or parsley to your recipes. One Fight the Fat member passed on herbs and chose to grow horseradish instead! "It's a root, and it's as easy to grow as a weed—that's my style of gardening. But easy or not, there's such satisfaction in eating something you yourself have grown. It must be connected to a basic instinct. I clean it and grate it and mix it with different fruit jellies

(I got the recipe from a Fight the Fat handout). When my very skinny and very picky sister-in-law came to dinner last July 4, I used it to spice up the fish…she asked for seconds, and the recipe!"

Chapter Six: Mid-diet Slump!

"If I believe I cannot do something, it makes me incapable of doing it.
But when I believe I can, then I acquire the ability to do it, even if
I did not have the ability in the beginning."
—Mahatma Gandhi

Middles don't have the excitement of beginnings or ends! Dr. Pepper commercials used to tell you that you needed a Dr. Pepper twice a day—for your mid-morning slump and your mid-afternoon down in the dump! There's midlife crisis and middle-age spread, and in Medieval times they even talked about a special demon that stalked you in the middle of the day, the Demon of the Afternoon (*Demon Meridianus*). All the other demons attacked you at night, but this one would pluck at your sleeve when you were feeling discouraged or tired in the middle of your work. I guess they suffered from the "mid" slump even then. He'd whisper in your ear *Give up!*

Most Fight the Fat members get a visit from this demon at about week six. Fight the Fat organizer Dianna Kirkwood says, "It's about now that your sweet tooth is beginning to ache. You're missing your old way of eating and forgetting the pain it caused—how angry you felt with yourself after bingeing on junk food, the lethargy and discomfort. You forget all the clothes you couldn't wear. You're forgetting all the things you couldn't do because of your weight.

"The first thing is to realize that the mid-diet slump is normal; it's a part of the whole process. By week six, it starts to sink in that you are leaving behind your old way of eating *for good*. The reality starts to hit you. Discouraging thoughts begin to cross your mind—and that's natural. It doesn't mean it's the end. *It's okay to feel discouraged.* Feelings come and go.

It's what you *do* about them that counts. Success is just around the corner, I keep telling myself: Don't quit! Just don't give in!"

The most important thing to remember is that *you're not alone; you have your team to turn to.* As feisty fat-fighter Sara says of her eight woman *Cascade* team, "Oh, whenever we feel that we are running out of steam, we do something together! Sometimes we've gone overnight to a hotel for a girls' night out, or we have a night of dancing, or we might just go out for supper together. We went to a play a few times; we went up to Minneapolis— our group sticks together because we just like each other..."

Another positive move you can make is to review your journal at this point in Fight the Fat—that's the payoff for all the writing or taping you've been doing. It's a way of *really* remembering how you felt in the beginning, of getting into the mindset you had when you started and of seeing how much you've changed. Take the time to really think about why you joined Fight the Fat (or bought this book!) and what this last month and a half has meant to you.

Fight the Fat organizer Jane Clemen says, "The danger doesn't come from the slump as much as it does from the feelings that come with it. We put pressure on ourselves to be exactly on target, and if we get off track a little, we feel as if everything's over. So, we quit, when if we just held on a little longer, we'd reap the rewards of all our work. It's human to slump a little. Progress isn't a straight line. Remember, if you take two steps forward and one backward, you're still a step ahead!"

The team *No More Flab*, a sturdy group of ten walkers, runners, and bikers from Dubuque, understands how important it is to look at progress this way. They put up the following poster and quotes in their meeting room— it's a great model to keep in mind.

"If you think you are defeated, you are.
If you think you can't, you don't.
If you like to win but think you can't
It's almost certain that you won't.

Life's battles don't always go
To the stronger woman or man.
But sooner or later, those who win
Are those who think they can!"
—The motto that golfer Arnold Palmer keeps on the wall of his office

On Persistence

Activity	Age
Failed in business	22
Ran for legislature—defeated	23
Failed in business…again	24
Elected to legislature	25
Sweetheart died	26
Suffered nervous breakdown	27
Defeated for speaker of the house	29
Defeated for nomination for congress	34
Elected to congress	37
Lost renomination	39
Defeated for senate	46
Defeated for nomination for vice president	47
Defeated for senate…again	49
Elected president of the United States	51

Who was he? Abe Lincoln!

"I'm a slow walker—but I never walk back."
—Abe Lincoln

"The best thing about the future is that it comes only one day at a time."
—Abe Lincoln

Lincoln's life is so inspiring since we can see now, from the distance of time, that his setbacks were part of the whole picture. His progress was anything but a straight line. Yet he did not give up despite his failures—and it was his belief in himself that allowed him to triumph.

As Bobbi Schell says, "The mind can be a weapon we use against ourselves. *What's the point!* we say after eating some chocolate or missing an exercise class. *You won't lose this week, so you might as well really enjoy yourself, have another!* That way of thinking can really make you crazy, and I'm sure it's familiar to anyone with a weight issue. But the mind can also be our best friend, focusing instead on inspiring thoughts and valuable insights."

Virginia is a perfect example of Bobbi's warning. She's done pretty well during her first Fight the Fat (fourteen pounds), but during her second Fight the Fat, after losing another nine pounds, she began to slump. She found herself cutting corners when it came to exercising. At first she skipped exercise classes, and then, during one hectic week, stopped exercising for a week even at home.

"I had too much to do that week. I work in Dubuque in a florist shop and we had two weddings and a convention at the same time. I had to put in a lot of overtime, but *every day of that week* I thought of something one of my teammates had read somewhere, *If you can't make the time to be healthy you better leave yourself plenty of time to be sick!*

"So, finally I went back to the gym and picked up where I'd left off. There's another good Fight the Fat saying (once you go through the ten-week campaign you're never the same afterwards. You hear so much good stuff!) I try to live by it. *It is the greatest of all mistakes to do nothing because you can only do a little. Do what you can.* I don't remember who said it..." (later, Dianna Kirkwood supplied the name of the author: Sydney Smith, 1771, clergyman and writer).

"But I stuck to that idea—*Do what you can!* That's how things really have changed for me now for the first time in all the years I've been struggling with my weight. Fight the Fat gave me the freedom to say, *Yeah, I've skipped exercise this week but that doesn't mean I have to eat. It doesn't have to be all or nothing. One meal, even one week isn't the whole ball game.* I had to accept the fact that I'm not perfect—that no one's perfect."

In other words, if you've fallen off a little by week six it's no big deal. What's important is that you are still with Fight the Fat. You are still hanging in there trying. And that's something that should be a source of satisfaction and pride.

Make week six a time to acknowledge this victory! You've had scores of victories since you joined, small ones and large ones, but it is easy to overlook them in your rush toward the finish. Remember, it is just as important to *realize where you're coming from as to keep you're eye on where you're going!*

Some people never understand how *empowering* it is to focus on what they have achieved. They are always worrying about how much more they have to do. But there's a huge boost that comes from realizing, *Hey, I can do five sit-ups and when I started I could barely do one.* Or, *Look at that! It's been six weeks and those stress techniques must really be kicking in—I feel so much calmer.*

Marie, another Fight the Fat participant, says, "I used to love being out in the fields when I was a kid and lived on the farm. I always did the disking—" (she explained that meant breaking up the large clods of earth after plowing). "I'd love just sitting on a tractor and going back and forth over the upturned soil. It made me feel so good—I'd think about it and miss it every spring.

"Then during a meeting I got to talking with my teammates and one of them said, *You know you don't have to have an excuse to get out in the fields. Just make the time and go there, woman!* I know this will sound silly, but I'd just never thought of that before. I'm really busy with my grandchildren and my husband is sick and needs my help. But now I make sure to do that a few times a month—even in the winter."

Marie's new habit isn't a success she can measure right away. It doesn't add up in terms of pounds lost. But, it's just as important, and it's the kind of success that will help keep Marie going—especially when she hits a plateau that may come about now (or that may come somewhat later, like after week ten; it depends on the individual).

You hit a plateau when your weight loss begins to slow down after that "big loss" during the first weeks. Your body adjusts to the new level of activity and the new eating pattern, and you can go for a long time without losing a single pound. Webster's dictionary defines a plateau as "an elevated track of level land." If you want a visual aid, picture yourself walking across a vast, arid desert. You're in a hurry to get across, but don't forget that along the way you're learning how to survive, you're gaining stamina, and you're becoming stronger.

Vona, who crossed many plateaus on her way to a forty-pound weight loss and a healthier life, says, "I refuse, I just refuse, to let the scale tell me how I should feel about myself. Sure, I weigh in because the scale can be a reality-check. I use it to make sure I'm not way off track. If I started gaining every week, of course I'd have to figure out what I was doing wrong. The scale can fib on a weekly basis—sometimes you hold water, sometimes you've been eating a lot of roughage—but over a period of weeks it won't lie. It's not a part of my routine I put much emphasis on, though. I know even before I step on a scale exactly how I'm doing. Being on the third notch of my belt or the second can tell me just as much.

"What I do care about, though," she continued, "is staying in control. I celebrate each day I don't go off on a binge! I bought a huge calendar for my kitchen, and the row of gold stars for all my good days have come to mean more to me than the numbers on the scale. Just *not* gaining has become a victory. I know that sooner or later the weight loss will come—it has already. I've lost forty pounds, though I have to lose more. My job isn't to worry about how fast the rest will be gone. I just have to do my part; I just have to stick to healthy guidelines and I know I'll be okay."

Fight the Fat member Judy of New Vienna, who has kept off twenty-four pounds for the last *four years*, also worked with her mental attitude as a way to keep going. She didn't struggle with her impulse to quit—she just postponed it. "All during my first Fight the Fat I promised myself, I *swore* that would be *it* the moment week ten was finished!

"And I meant it; I counted the days until week ten. *If I pull out when week ten comes around, I'll have finished it. I won't be a quitter,* I told myself. *I won't be letting down my team.* But when week ten came 'round I felt so proud of myself for having come so far...that I kind of kept going. Now I've completed four Fight the Fat campaigns and I'm still planning to quit—someday. But I have a feeling it won't be soon!"

Another positive step you can take to combat your throw-in-the-towel blues is to rethink your exercise program. Mercy's Supervisor of Rehabilitation Outreach Services Bobbi Schell, says, "Members have to really *listen* to their bodies if they're going to make exercise a regular part of their lives. You don't automatically know what you can do. It's not just a matter of finding out what your heart rate is! You have to enjoy what you're doing, you have to get just the right mix of developing your muscles, increasing your strength and endurance, and taking pleasure in what you're doing. If you don't look forward to your exercise sessions, if you groan and moan about them, you're not going to keep it up!"

Whatever the exercise you're doing, Bobbi advises people to *start slow,* and don't forget, if your goal is a healthy *life,* week six of Fight the Fat is just the beginning! Ask yourself, are you exercising at a smart rate, or have you taken on too much? "So many people start out by throwing themselves into a grueling routine," Bobbi warns. "They are determined to get fit in a hurry, and a few weeks later they've given up. The exercise bikes are in the attic and they're back on the couch. They can't sustain it. You have to develop a routine you can maintain over a lifetime, you have to ease into it. Of course it's good to be challenged, to work up a sweat and get your heart pumping...but if you do too much too soon, you'll burn out."

Fight the Fat member Joyce took Bobbi's advice, and, during her first Fight the Fat, discovered what her own needs were. "I'd gone up and down for years, but this time I had no choice but to succeed," she told me during a break at the Dyersville Hardee's where she works. "My extra weight had been affecting my heart. I have fibrillations and there were other complications because of it. Fight the Fat came along at just the right time for me.

"During the week I walk to work three miles back and forth. My goal was to walk at least twice a week. If I walk more, five times, for example, my feet start to hurt since I'm standing all day. I also found out that at night, when I used to do my worst overeating, if I just go out at the spur of the moment for fifteen or twenty minutes it relaxes me. After dinner or when I'm in the mood for a snack, I just walk long enough to put myself in a good mood. That's really helped me cut down on nighttime eating, and I sleep better too because of it."

By "listening" to her body, Joyce discovered her own pattern and she stuck to walking over a long period of time. If she'd overdone it, her walking plan wouldn't have lasted long enough for her to wear out her first pair of walking shoes!

Sometimes the opposite is true—you may have to *add* another activity, or discover a new healthy habit, or seek out a new person who can be an additional source of support. You can use your journal as a way of figuring out what you need. Too often, people blindly react to feelings. *I'm depressed; if I eat I'll feel better. That's the way I've always handled it. Okay, where's the nearest bakery?* Use the journal to break this pattern and think things out instead. *Am I doing too much or too little? Do I feel guilty or sorry for myself? Do I feel unable to cope, or am I afraid of success?*

Of course, success can be frightening. As Bill Cosby says, "You have to decide that you want it more than you are afraid of it." There are all kinds of anxieties accompanying change that you might not be aware of. "What might be causing your slump now is that you are entering into a high-risk zone," says Dianna Kirkwood, who has watched many members go through a metamorphosis. "You are on the brink of becoming the new you! For someone hiding behind layers of fat for years, that idea can be frightening as well as inspiring. I have seen members who have shed a great deal of weight still walking or getting up from a chair the way they used to. They're not yet comfortable with their new bodies. Their mind hasn't caught up with reality—yet. But give it time. Trust me. It does."

But by week six, the new bodies are still in the future—a scary, inspiring possibility. "When you're not *there* yet you really need somebody to notice," says Jan of New Vienna. "It's not dramatic yet. I mean, if you've lost seven or eight pounds and have thirty more to go, it's easy for people to overlook what you've done. And that makes you yourself overlook it."

That is why Fight the Fat is constantly having its members pay attention to the so-called *small* changes that lay the groundwork for the new you. A Fight the Fat handout for meeting number six puts it this way, "When the Greek engineer Archimedes claimed that he could move the world, he was referring to the use of levers. We all have many tools at our disposal to change our world. One of the most important is our attitude. When asked, *Can you lift a ton?*, most folks would say *No!* This is because we are geared to the large goal, not the steps by which we reach it. Walk up one flight of stairs and you have lifted a ton, step by small step!"

Reaching week six is in some ways like being a teenager who is not a kid anymore and not yet an adult. Like a teenager, you have to find yourself; like a teenager, you suffer from growing pains. Your new habits are not yet second nature, and your old habits are still with you. You're unsure of where you're going, and you keep looking around, secretly longing for the past!

Cindy joined Fight the Fat on a dare from her daughter (*"I'll quit smoking if you lose weight!"*). She had been exercising steadily until she got a bad case of mid-diet slump and started taking off days "to relax."

"By this point [she was in week seven], you're exercising but not enjoying it as much as you were before. The novelty has worn off. And you're not enjoying it as much as people who are already fit. It's hard to drag yourself out for a walk when you're like me—thirty-nine pounds overweight. It's more work for me to get on a treadmill than it is for my daughter to do it. The stage I'm at reminds me of when I started taking piano in elementary school: I knew enough to do the exercises but I couldn't yet play the songs, which was the real fun."

Cindy may be exaggerating a little (self-pity creeps in and makes you do that!), but it's true that she can't *yet* do her exercises with as much ease as she'd like. "The key word here is *yet*," says Mercy's Supervisor of Rehabilitation Outreach Services Bobbi Schell, who exercises *with ease* although she is still some eighty pounds above her weight goal. Just watching her move, her body tone, and the joy it gives her to reach and stretch and jump is inspiring. "If Cindy keeps on exercising she'll be able to get on the treadmill with all the ease in the world. But if she's looking for an excuse to quit, she'll find many—she doesn't have to blame exercise!" she laughs. "Believe me, there are hundreds of reasons. And I've heard them all!"

"Such as?" I asked, curious.

"Such as—*I got a cold and quit! Not eating enough was lowering my immunity!* [Of course, exercise helps strengthen the immune system while sugar compromises it.]

"*I couldn't sleep—and I can't afford to have insomnia since I have to be alert at work. So, I got up at midnight and finished off a chocolate cake!* [Of course, exercise will help give you a good night sleep.]

"*It's cold out, and if I don't eat enough my fingers and toes freeze. I have poor circulation. So, I went back to pie a la mode as a snack!* [Of course, pie a la mode means ice cream! And isn't ice cream *cold*? Exercise is a good way to improve the circulation *naturally*. A few sit-ups and push-ups would have done this woman more good than all that sugar!]

"The point is, if anyone says it's hard for them to exercise *that means it's hard for them to move. Period.* And the more sedentary they become, the worse it will get. Being out of shape is *not* a reason to quit—it's a reason to try even harder. Let's be honest—*at least with ourselves!*"

Visiting Bobbi Schell's exercise class in Cascade, this dynamic woman makes you aware of what is possible, regardless of whether it's week six or week sixty. She and her team members have exercised together for months, and by now they've gotten to the point where they can show up tired and out of sorts individually, yet by working together, generate megawatts of team energy.

Bobbi herself has had a hard day helping patients, attending hospital meetings, and dealing with family needs. Meeting her earlier in the gym's office, I thought she looked a little harried as she made some last minute calls. But now she is a different person.

"I'm too fat—I can't do it," I overhear a teammate complain. Bobbi shows her how to do a modified form of the exercise—a push-up against the wall. She seems to be aglow with enthusiasm and ready to take nothing but total health.

"Come on!" she sings out to her teammates. "Let's get with it! Let's get moving! Let's get going! Turn your instant calorie burner *on!*" She pushes a button and the theme song from *Rocky* echoes throughout the gym. "When you start giving your body the exercise it needs and the right foods it needs, you don't have to sit thinking about weight loss all the time. It's a natural, automatic outcome! Let's go!"

And you know what, they do!

The week six meeting of the Dyersville Fight the Fat ended with an exclamation mark! Fight the Fat organizer Dianna Kirkwood summed up the challenge presented by this mid-point in the campaign. "I know many of you are feeling that it's getting hard around now. Many of you are struggling. But think of this week as a chance to grow, to dig your heels in and fight—after all, we Iowans are known for our stubbornness!

"A Fight the Fat speaker told us last year that the Chinese word for *crisis* is also *opportunity*—and that's a good thing to keep in mind this week! The fact that we are struggling is good! We were *meant* to struggle—and to win! Take the struggle out of life and what would it be? A philosopher once wrote, *What doesn't kill you makes you stronger!* The next time you feel discouraged and pushed to your limit, remember the words of a well-known American speaker, Napoleon Hill, 'The strongest oak tree is not the one that is protected from the storm and hidden from the sun. It's the one that stands in the open where it is compelled to struggle for its existence against the winds and rains and the scorching sun!'

"Yes, you're tempted. Yes, now things get harder—week six is reality! But remember, whether it will be a slump or a milestone is up to you!"

Your Workbook

The Bulletin Board

"The greater part of our happiness or misery depends on our dispositions and not on our circumstances. We carry the seeds of the one or the other about with us in our minds wherever we go."
—Martha Washington

"Character is fate."
—Greek saying

"The only people who achieve much are those who do so while the conditions are still unfavorable. Favorable conditions never come."
—C.S. Lewis

"Start by doing what's necessary, then what's possible, and suddenly you are doing the impossible."
—St Francis of Assisi

In a survey of participants following the May 2000 completion of the ten-week Fight the Fat in Dyersville, 112 people responded with this information:

- 71 percent had lost ten or more pounds.
- 78 percent agreed strongly that Fight the Fat increased their knowledge of healthy eating habits.

For Your Bulletin Board

For those who like statistics, here's the lowdown on the Iowa Fight the Fat campaigns.

Fight the Fat Fact Sheet

Fight the Fat in Dyersville, Iowa:
March–June 1998: 383 participants lost 3,998 pounds
January–March 1999: 452 participants lost 3,559 pounds
March–May 2000: 272 participants lost 2,785 pounds
March–May 2001: 183 participants lost 1,776 pounds

Fight the Fat in Dubuque, Iowa:
February–April 2001: 505 participants lost 3,911 pounds

Fight the Fat in Monticello, Iowa:
October–December 1999: 205 participants lost 1,554 pounds

Fight the Fat in Elkader, Iowa:
March–May 2000: 109 participants lost 943 pounds
March–May 2001: 140 participants lost 842 pounds

Your Journal

"The best way to get rid of a bad habit is to replace it with a good one!" advises Ray, Fight the Fat member who lost thirty-four pounds and now jogs four times a week. "I look forward to my jog now the way I used to look forward to a whole pizza with pepperoni washed down with beer!"

1) *Describe three self-destructive habits you want to replace with three healthy habits.*
2) *What concrete steps must you take to achieve this change?*

Healthy Habit for the Week

Straighten up! The foremost expert on back pain in this country, Dr. Leon Root, the author of *Oh, My Aching Back,* states that he never treated a patient who had good posture. Good posture not only improves your walking form, which means you'll burn up more fat, but it also makes you look better, more fit, and slimmer right away. You lose pounds just by straightening up!

Marilu Henner, author of *Total Health Makeover, Ten Steps To Your Best Body,* says, "As a dancer, one of the most important things I strive for is *finding my center...*The way you carry your body (your posture) speaks volumes about the balance you have in your life. If you were to look at yourself from a side view, imagine seeing a line that runs down the center of your body. What is in front of that line should be equal to what is behind that line...If your posture is slouchy and distorted, something is out of balance." So, straighten up!

Reward for the Week

You are back in caveman times! You make a kill—but you have to devour it quickly because at any moment another, stronger predator can show up on the plain and take away your meal. Or, you drag your kill back to the cave. There in the darkness that spells security, you linger over your meal for hours, perhaps days.

These ancient patterns are not so different in terms of fast food restaurants (eating quickly, out in the "open field") and pricey, gourmet restaurants (eating in your cave)! The whole atmosphere of those bright diners and fast food joints gives your brain the unconscious message *Rush! Get it over with.* Perhaps some primal memory is triggered. Who knows? But, for whatever reason, in those places you are in and out.

The opposite is true of the upscale restaurants where they want you to linger, to order an extra expensive side dish, perhaps, or a bottle of wine— where the eating goes on, cave-style, for hours.

So, for your reward this week, *relax* in that cave of yours with a meal that is as pleasing to the eye as it is to the palate. Arrange flowers, bring out the china you reserve for company—be your own guest without the stress of having any other guests. Honor yourself with scented candles, soft music, silk dinner napkins, the works. And apart from your one special meal, try to include some element of elegance and beauty at every meal during the week, whether it's flowers or just the way the food is arranged. Restaurateurs understand how important atmosphere is psychologically…remember, so much of eating goes on in the head.

Team Activity for the Week

You've heard of wine-tasting festivals? Well, this week your team will create a food-tasting hour, complete with all the healthy suggestions you can come up with. This ensures that you *act* on what you've been talking about since *action* is the key to success in Fight the Fat. Use foods of the week, use recipes you make up yourself or have heard about—you don't have to bring in entire meals for everyone. The idea is to taste and inspire others!

A member of the *No More 2 Fat Blues* brought in a great pumpkin pie. After giving the recipe, she read the following fact she had clipped from *Prevention Magazine.*

"Studies show that the aroma of pumpkin pie can increase penile blood flow by 40 percent."

She went on to give this healthy version of the pie that she got from Jane Clemen of Fight the Fat. (You can be sure that all her teammates were busily copying it down—since the dish was rich in beta-carotene and fiber, of course!)

Crunchy Crust Light Pumpkin Pie

Crust

2 tbsp. melted margarine

1 egg white

⅔ cup whole wheat flour

¼ cup brown sugar

1) Combine crust ingredients and mix well.
2) Firmly press mixture onto bottom and sides of a 9-inch pie plate sprayed with non-stick cooking spray.

Filling

2 eggs

1 16-ounce can pumpkin

½ cup sugar

¼ tsp. salt

1 tsp. cinnamon

½ tsp. ginger

¼ tsp. ground cloves

1⅔ cups fat-free evaporated milk (12-ounce can)

1) Beat eggs slightly with a rotary beater.
2) Beat in remaining ingredients.
3) Pour into pie pan.
4) Bake for 15 minutes at 425º F.
5) Reduce oven temperature to 350º F and bake 45 minutes longer or until a knife inserted in the center comes out clean.

(212 calories, 4.6 grams fat)

Another, even less fattening option is the following Pumpkin Custard Pie recipe, courtesy of Jennifer Raymond, author of *The Peaceful Palate* and *Fat-free & Easy* published by Heart & Soul Publishing.

Pumpkin Custard Pie

1 9-inch pie crust (see following recipe)

½ cup sugar or other sweetener

4 tbsp. cornstarch

1 tsp. cinnamon

½ tsp. ginger

⅛ tsp. cloves

½ tsp. salt

1 15-ounce can solid-pack pumpkin

1½ cups soy milk or rice milk

1) Preheat the oven to 350 F.

2) In a large bowl, stir together the sugar, cornstarch, spices, and salt.

3) Blend in the pumpkin and milk, then pour into a 9-inch crust.

4) Bake until set, about 45 minutes.

5) Cool before cutting.

Serve while wearing a black negligee! Enjoy!

(150 calories, 0 grams fat)

Fat-free Pie Crust

1 cup Grape-Nuts cereal

¼ cup apple juice concentrate (undiluted)

1) Preheat oven to 350º F.

2) Mix ingredients and pat into a 9-inch pan.

3) Bake for 8 minutes.

(68 calories, 0 grams fat)

Golden Rule for the Week

"To lengthen thy life, lessen thy meals!"
—Ben Franklin

Change *lessen* to *lighten* and Fight the Fat agrees, old Ben got it right! Strategy: keep eating during the day! Cut back at night! Small frequent snacks or meals are the key. Those huge twenty-course feasts might have been great in Roman days but hey, you don't want to look like Nero!

Jennifer, a Fight the Fat success story, focused on the *when* of eating. "My old pattern was to go from lunch to dinner without eating—I was trying to *be good*—that's how I thought of it. No snacking between meals. I'd come home all bloated up with diet soda and then have my main meal of the day. I was entitled to it, I felt, but afterwards I always felt tired. Then one of the team captains at Fight the Fat asked how many people ate their main meal at night and what they did after that? It turned out that most of us watched some television, or sat around and talked before going to sleep. So, she asked us why don't we try to switch that eating up to the daytime when we are burning up calories, and her suggestion made sense.

"Now I *break up* my big evening meal—I take some of it with me to work. I'll have a baked potato at eleven in the morning, for example, or I'll have the soup as a pick-me-up in the middle of the afternoon. Sometimes I'll even have the steak or chicken for lunch and try to keep the nighttime eating lighter—salad with some bread and fruit. I even exercise a little after dinner. I don't do more than ten or fifteen minutes at night, but I know I feel better from it. This new eating schedule is what really got me started. It was a major factor."

Some Good Snack Ideas
- Apple wedges spread with peanut butter (measure the peanut butter by the teaspoon).

- Whole-grain muffins (weigh the muffins, portion sizes keep getting bigger in the good old overweight USA).
- Whole wheat sesame bread sticks.
- Nonfat or low-fat yogurt topped with wheat germ, raisins (measure!), or fresh fruit.

Although you may not want to plan *all* your snacks in advance, this week try it and see how it affects your eating. Sit down and come up with ideas for the week and make sure that you'll have the food you need for each one in advance. Advance planning is crucial since our society has made it so easy to go for foods loaded with fat and sugar and low in nutritional value (a stop off at the mall to buy a pair of shoes can net you two days worth of calories before you know it!).

How many times have you grabbed some junk food *you might not even have wanted* because nothing else was available? Margaret, a Fight the Fat member, says, "If I'm on the road and feeling hungry—driving always does it to me—I don't tell myself *You've already had lunch. Forget it.* Because I know if I do that, the next time I make a ladies room stop, I'll be eating a double cheeseburger. Instead, the car is loaded with healthy snacks; I could open up a supermarket. A low-fat, whole wheat bread, turkey sandwich and cut-up vegetables keep me from going crazy. As a precaution, I also always bring snacks to work. That way I can eat something in the car on the way home. I never come home starving the way I used to."

Louise, another Fight the Fat member, has this to add, "I don't let myself get hungry anymore. I've discovered that when people ask me to try a piece of cake they've just made or to go for ice cream with them, it's easier to say *no* if I'm not hungry. I say it like I mean it, and people usually leave me alone after that."

Food of the Week

Be rich—in *beta-carotene!*
Be food smart!
Be healthy!

Many studies over the years have shown that foods like *carrots, pumpkins,* and *yams*—sweet potatoes, red peppers, butternut squash, and spinach (and all other dark leafy green vegetables)—lower the risk of heart disease and cancer. Such foods are stored by the body as vitamin A, which is good for the vision and strengthens the immune system. An additional payoff is healthier skin! One example of a creative, low-calorie and health promoting addition to your meal is the Curried Carrot soup. The strong flavor will please your palette, sending your brain the message, "I'm satisfied," while the nutritional benefits will keep you healthy. What more can you ask? Here are two fun to eat, delicious, carotene-rich recipes:

Thai Sweet Potatoes Over Rice

1½ pounds sweet potatoes, peeled and cut into ½-inch pieces
1 tbsp. vegetable oil
1 onion, chopped
2 cloves garlic, minced
1½ tbsp. fresh grated gingerroot
2 tsp curry powder
⅛ to ¼ tsp crushed red pepper flakes
1 can (12 oz.) evaporated skim milk
½ tsp coconut extract
½ cup water
½ tsp (or less) Light Salt
1 cup frozen green peas, thawed
1 tbsp. grated lemon peel
4 cups hot, cooked basmati or other white rice

2 tbsp. unsalted dry-roasted peanuts
¼ cup chopped fresh cilantro

1) In a large saucepan, cover the sweet potatoes with water and heat until boiling.
2) Cool 10 minutes; drain and set aside.
3) In a large skillet, heat the oil; add the onion and sauté until tender. Add the garlic, ginger, curry powder, and pepper flakes; cook, stirring occasionally, three minutes.
4) Add the cooked sweet potatoes, evaporated milk, coconut extract, water, and Light Salt. Heat to boiling.
5) Reduce the heat, cover, and simmer for 20 minutes or until the potatoes are tender.
6) Remove from the heat and stir in the peas and lemon peel. Place the hot, cooked rice in a serving dish and top with the potato mixture.
7) Sprinkle with peanuts and cilantro and serve. Serves six.

(400 calories, 5 grams fat)

(From *The New American Diet Cookbook* by Sonja L. Connor and William E. Connor, which has 250+ healthy recipes including large sections on beans, seafood, and soups.)

Curried Carrot Soup
1 tbsp. olive oil
2 cups diced onion
½ cup diced celery
1 tsp curry powder (or to taste)
4 cups finely sliced carrots
1½ cups diced potatoes
3 cups water
Salt and pepper (to taste)

1 tbsp. sugar

8 tbsp. low-fat, plain yogurt

Parsley

1) Heat oil in a saucepan. Add celery and onion and cook until softened.

2) Sprinkle with curry powder; cook and stir.

3) Add potatoes, carrots, water, salt, and pepper; stir.

4) Cover and bring to a boil; reduce heat and simmer about a half-hour.

5) Puree. Return to pot, stirring in sugar and reheat.

6) Add 1½ tbsp. of yogurt per bowl and a sprinkling of parsley.

Makes 5 servings.

(130 calories, 4 grams fat)

Another Beta-carotene Boost

In the "dark green leafy" department, people may be unfamiliar with kale, so, we have included some information about how to prepare it.

Kale. It doesn't get healthier than this! This is a terrific leafy green vegetable from the cabbage family. Wash thoroughly and rinse. Dry as much as possible. Shake off excess water. Cut up into small lengths, about four inches long. The best pot to cook it in is a wok heated with a little olive or canola oil. Chop up garlic and put it into the heated wok first. Stir for a few seconds for flavor; add kale and stir-fry until it wilts a little (about five minutes). Toss kale in the oil for a minute and add a pinch or two of salt together with a little (about a tablespoon) of cooking wine or water for one large bunch of kale. Let it cook again for another couple of minutes. (Optional: add soy sauce to taste.) Very rich in minerals, one ounce of kale provides 38 milligrams of calcium.

Self-empowerment Exercise for the Week

Nancy Reagan had an anti-drug campaign whose slogan was *Just say no!* Many overweight people are *terrible* at saying *no!* They give in to every request from children, friends, and neighbors, and end up having no time for their own needs. They eat to give themselves what they need.

Rosalie Kaufman, author of *Yes You Can!* and prize-winning Weight Watchers® group leader, says, "*A bankrupt person cannot give anything to anyone!* Learn how to protect your time: you need it to calm down from stress, to exercise, [and] to carefully prepare healthy meals for yourself."

There are courses in self-assertiveness training and books and tapes that you can study with your teammates. You may find such a course useful, or you may decide to work through this problem with your Fight the Fat buddy, comparing notes and discussing effective strategies. Such situations can include food-related problems like going out to eat with friends that are set on picking a restaurant that you know is not good for you. Or they can be non-food situations where you have to learn to be firm while being polite.

Go through a whole range of possible responses from the person you are refusing/confronting and take note of your responses and your feelings. Focus on situations that you feel have led to out of control eating in the past.

Don't be a victim. You can make changes in your life only if you take responsibility for your actions.

Look at the Difference

I couldn't exercise because I had to give my neighbor a lift to work all week—her car broke down. She's been so wonderful to me that I just had to help her out when she asked me. She's such a good person and she's always there for me.

I ended up putting on some weight this week and I got discouraged and dropped out. What's the use of all this hard work if I'm going to end up gaining weight? I'll never lose enough for it to make a difference. I have so much to do and I feel so bad without my favorite desserts anyway! What can I do?

Scenario #2

Tell yourself—*I'm at a crossroads in my life. It's now or never. I've been carrying around too much weight and it's been affecting my mood, my health, and my ability to function. If I don't do something about it, it will only get worse. I have to make this my priority. Nothing can get in the way. Others may need me for "X," "Y," or "Z," but they will survive. They will get through it. My exercise or my food preparation time is sacred for me. Also, since I know that on some level I am resisting this change, let me remember that it is easier for me to give up my time to somebody else than it is to look myself straight in the mirror and say: you will change! You will become active, thin, and fit!*

"I'm sorry, I wish I could, but I can't help you this week. I just can't." Helping others is good, but taking care of you is essential!

Stress Antidote for the Week

Note: since a pet is *not* for everyone, alternative stress antidotes for the week are given below.

I want to strive to become the person my dog thinks I am.

Wendy adopted a dog—or it adopted her. "I thought of something I read in a Fight the Fat handout," she said. *"How about taking your dog out for a long walk or run? You won't regret it. A dog is the only being on earth that loves you more than he loves himself.*—Josh Billings.

"I figured on those cold wet Sunday mornings, he'll be all over me and raring to go—no more sleeping in."

If you can't take in a dog, another good idea is to offer to regularly walk the dog of a neighbor or friend. After all, as Andrew Rooney says, "The average dog is a nicer person than the average person!"

Studies have shown that having a pet to come home to (that wagging tail, those joyful yelps) lowers blood pressure (and this includes having purring cats to stroke).

Many organizations work with nursing homes and regularly bring dogs to the elderly as therapy. The animal's presence is healing.

Your dog or your cat is a great listener. As Chris Morley puts it, "No one appreciates the very special genius of your conversation as your dog does!"

Researchers at Indiana University asked thirty couples to discuss marital conflicts in sessions with and without their pet dogs. Sessions were videotaped and the couples' physical responses recorded. Findings: "The dog's presence had a soothing effect on measured physical responses in all the cases. The presence of the dog was associated with changes in the emotional and physiological climate that are favorable for the process of marital conflict resolution."

If you haven't given yourself the pleasure of owning a pet because you work long hours and feel that it's unfair to the animal, you might want to rethink your decision. Check out the pet sitters in your region in the yellow pages—they may be the backup you need. For example, there's Yuppie Puppie in New York City, Pet Companions in Somerville, Massachusetts, and the All Dogs Gym in Manchester, New Hampshire.

Finally, in choosing a pet—cat, dog, bird, or smaller creature, such as a hamster or rabbit—make sure you consider whether he will do well in the home you provide for him. Size isn't always the deciding factor. Great Danes, for example, are happy in an apartment if they get regular exercise, while active dogs like retrievers don't do well in small living quarters without a place to run. Whatever your choice, an animal is a wonderful, *non-caloric* way of bringing joy and fun into your life!

Some Alternative Suggestions for Week Six

Thinking Games. Why are crossword puzzles and solitaire so popular? They allow you a "mini-vacation" right where you are. You get away from everything, all those pressures nagging at you, for a half-hour "trip." Used regularly, these fun, non-food stress relievers can do the trick when you start craving. And as your skill increases and you start graduating to more complicated puzzles or forms of solitaire (there are books explaining intricate solitaire patterns), you will not even notice that you are solving the willpower puzzle as well!

Cook! Have you ever found that after cooking a big meal you are less hungry? That is because the odors of the cooking send signals to our brain. You are being nourished! The whole process is a loving and self-nurturing one. You are not sneaking a chocolate bar when no one is looking and gobbling it down to an inner chorus of guilt! You are dealing with food in a careful and considered way: it is not the forbidden, hidden sin! You are taking time to make the meal you need and deserve!

Of course, sometimes you have to buy meals ready-made. You can do that also—you can depend on Lean Cuisine or the frozen Weight Watchers® meals to get you through a day. But what is more relaxing and luxurious than preparing a sumptuous meal or even just a dessert or a superb dish?

There is nothing like a good book. Author Elizabeth Hardwick is eloquent on the subject, "The greatest gift is a passion for reading. It is cheap; it consoles; it distracts; it excites; it gives you knowledge of the world and experience of a wide kind. It is a moral illumination." Not only is reading a wonderful way "out" when you are feeling stressed, but it's also free and a great habit to get the kids into. When they're nagging at you and you're at the end of your patience, take them to a library instead of a mall. While they're busy in the kids' section, you can browse the biographies, the mysteries, or the inspirational section! Libraries, big chain stores, and many independent booksellers have regularly scheduled events in which writers read from their own works and after which there are question-and-answer periods. Not only will such events take your mind off everything, but you will also broaden your perspectives. Calorie cost: a big fat *zero*!

Solitude. Too often, instead of realizing we need some time to recover from the day, we turn to food to calm us or quiet us down—when that hour alone would be a better solution. Remember, the word *recreation* means, literally, to recreate; we have to learn how to let go of some of the tensions and stresses that lead to overeating.

Chapter Seven: Glorious Food

"Food, glorious food!"
—*Oliver*, **Broadway Musical**

"You can't change everything at once. Just do it once and for all!"
—Fight the Fat slogan

The following story of how six members of the Dyersville team *The New Stars* interacted is an example of Fight the Fat at its best.

I heard about it while talking to Maxine, a member who'd lost eighteen pounds during the last year's Fight the Fat campaign. When I asked her how she was doing now, she told me that not only had she kept those eighteen pounds off, but she'd also lost an additional six since she'd started biking and power walking on alternate days. *And* she was doing all this while helping out with her three young grandchildren!

Impressed by her success, I asked her what the No. 1 lesson she'd learned from Fight the Fat was.

"That's easy," she laughed. "I learned that I really love food."

"What do you mean?" I said, startled.

"Just what I said! I guess it sounds kind of funny, but that's what's saved me. Being on a Fight the Fat team got me into food, all kinds of new foods. For one of our team projects, everyone had to taste at least two healthy foods we hadn't tried before and bring in a report.

"I wasn't very happy about the assignment—it was a busy week and I didn't feel like looking around for something new. But a friend I'd made on the team raved about tofu and invited me over to taste it the way she prepares it: tofu cut up into squares and topped with diced scallions and shredded ginger and soy sauce. She didn't even fry it. We ate it raw and I loved it this way. So, that was the beginning. I realized that if I was going to keep going, I'd have to begin to do something different, really different, from all the other times I failed at trying to lose weight.

"And now I'm into it—Japanese, Scandinavian, Ethiopian food, you name it. I especially like the way the Chinese eat fish. It's very simple, very healthy, and delicious. You can do fish in many different ways, but their basic technique is to slice thin strips of fresh ginger and chop up scallions, which you sprinkle on top of the fish and then steam it for about ten minutes, adding a little soy sauce when it's done. If Confucius had written a cookbook, this would have been his main recipe."

"That's pretty amazing! You're becoming a gourmet, Maxine."

"What I've come to realize is that if I want to stay thin, I have to eat—and eat—and eat well! I mean it really helps to become interested in food, to plan and get good recipes and think about your meals. Last year one of the Fight the Fat speakers was a gal from a small community just north of Dyersville. [She'd] written a book of delicious and simple recipes..." [M.J. Smith, *Five in Twenty*—recipes that require a maximum of five easy-to-find ingredients and can be prepared in no more than twenty minutes.] "She brought in a small grill and made them for us right there. So, I started slow, with some simple but good menus.

"Then dietician Jane Clemen said that most people don't really *taste* their food—they just bolt it down. Tasting takes place in the mouth, which really means the mind. It's your mind you have to satisfy. *Gourmet is the name for someone who appreciates fine food,* she said, *but gourmand is the French word for a pig!* I always connected the two, but I began to realize that they're as different as an alcoholic and a lover of fine wines.

"The more I thought about it, the more I realized it was true. I didn't take the time to taste my food! I just ate whatever was high in fat and sugar, and half the time I didn't really know what I was eating! It wasn't about enjoying different tastes or subtle flavors, it was about feeling stuffed or getting a sugar high and getting *blissed out.* I'm trying to get away from that now. My favorite magazine is *Food and Wine* these days. I'm learning new things all the time. It's awesome, the endless possibilities and combinations."

When I asked her for an example, she told me about Asian spices. She found them in Dubuque's Oriental Market—galangal (it has a sharp peppery flavor); tamarind (a sour pulp and seeds from a large pod); kaffir lime leaves (a lemon-lime flavor—the idea is to wrap the kaffir leaves, around scallops to give them an interesting, tart flavor. "Before Fight the Fat," she went on, "I stuck to cheeseburgers, milk shakes, and chocolate! In those days, if something was sweet or greasy, it was good. Now I've learned that even with everyday foods, you can always do *something*. Just listen to this, it's from the latest Fight the Fat handout. I put it up on my bulletin board. *Don't think of them as vegetables. Think of them as bursts of flavor! Here are some ideas for designer veggies: broccoli made cool with hot curry, marjoram, and a pinch of poppy seeds! Asparagus taking a bath in soy sauce, lemon juice, and sesame seeds! Cabbage made user-friendly with cider vinegar, chives, and caraway seeds. Summer squash needs to be enlivened—a dash of dill or oregano plus soy sauce can do it.*

"Now I'm developing a new standard when it comes to my taste buds. Sugar is no longer the ultimate, fat is no longer the be-all-and-the-end-all. And I like the adventure. I'll try anything at least once."

When I asked her how much time she spends on her meal preparation, she couldn't answer exactly—maybe because she finds it enjoyable. She used the weekends to plan for her coming week, finding that it made her look forward to her meals and gave her the feeling of being in control. She went through cookbooks and magazines and wrote down recipes and sometimes invited the team over to dinner. They all knew they'd be in for something different at her house. "Now that I've got all these Asian spices, this is what I'm going to make them next week," she chuckled, describing the following recipe:

Lemongrass Chicken

(Also good for salmon and scallops)

2 stalks fresh lemongrass, tender white inner bulbs only, smashed and coarsely chopped

2 large shallots, coarsely chopped (¼ pound)
2 garlic cloves, coarsely chopped
1 Thai chile, chopped
1 tbsp. Asian fish sauce
4 boneless chicken breast halves, (about 7 ounces each)
1 tbsp. vegetable oil
Salt and freshly ground pepper

1) In a food processor, combine the lemongrass with the shallots, garlic, chile, and fish sauce. Pulse to a coarse paste. Set the chicken
   breasts on a plate. Spread the paste on the fleshy side of the chicken,
   cover, and refrigerate for at least 2 hours. Bring the chicken to room
   temperature before cooking.
2) Preheat the oven to 450°. Transfer the chicken, skin side down, to
   paper towels. Heat the oil in a large nonstick ovenproof skillet.
3) Add the chicken, season with salt and pepper, and cook over moderately high heat until lightly browned on the bottom, about five
   minutes.
4) Transfer the skillet to the oven and roast the chicken for seven minutes, or until it is deep golden on the bottom. Carefully turn the
   chicken, season with salt and pepper, and roast for five minutes
   longer, or until cooked through.
5) Set the chicken breasts on a platter or plates and serve.
The lemongrass paste can be refrigerated for two days.

"That's the latest in *Food and Wine,*" she concluded.

"Your guests sound lucky!" I told her.

"Actually, I'm glad to cook for them! It keeps me on my toes. I know
they're expecting something *interesting* at my house and I don't want to dis-
appoint them."

Maxine's right on target as far as the nutrition experts are concerned.
Studies have shown that dieters who included a large range of foods in

their menus ended up maintaining their weight loss far better than those who stuck to a limited number of basic foods.

I asked Maxine's teammate, Sue, whether she'd ever been her guest and she answered with an exclamation: "You bet! Sometimes the food is great, and sometimes she makes dishes you *have to develop a taste for*, if you know what I mean. But it's *always fun* to go there because you're surprised."

When I asked Sue whether she'd used any of Maxine's ideas herself, she said, "Oh yes. For my husband's birthday, I made this meal, Indonesian rice, that had a zillion ingredients—you had to do a lot of shopping for it. But only *one* of them needed to be cooked—the rice. The rest you just mixed in. It was really good for the summer when you don't feel like cooking much. You also have to play around with the proportions and the ingredients till you get the flavor you want.

"For example, I like it sweeter, so I add extra currents and chunks of pineapple to the rice after mixing in chopped scallions, snow peas, cashews, diced peppers, onions, carrots, water chestnuts, and bamboo shoots. Don't ask me the proportions; that's something you have to work out to suit yourself. The sauce should be mostly orange juice to which you add soy sauce, a tablespoon of sesame oil, fresh garlic, fresh pepper, and fresh ginger. Shake it well—whatever's left over makes a good salad dressing. Pour on the sauce and let the mixture chill in the fridge overnight and serve with black bread and a light wine. You can add or subtract from the main ingredients. I know Maxine had many other vegetables she sliced and diced in. But you get the idea. It's a light, fun meal. And for dessert, she had something simple but also really nice. She cut up four plums into very, very thin wedges and left them to soak for about two hours in one-fourth cup fresh orange juice, one-half tablespoon sugar, and one tablespoon finely shredded fresh mint leaves. The plums were about eighty calories per serving with less than one gram of fat. The Indonesian Rice is your guess—nobody figured it out because it was kind of a party. But you won't get fat on it, I can promise you. I came in with a two pound loss that week!"

As I started to say good-bye, another team member (and neighbor), Julie, stopped by. A bright vivacious woman that helps out in her husband's dry goods store as well as taking care of two children, her face lit up with enthusiasm when she heard what we were talking about.

"The news isn't out yet," she confided, "but Maxine is giving a Hawaiian Luau soon! It's to celebrate the second anniversary of our team working together. She hasn't told me everything she's making, but she already gave me two new recipes, Hawaiian style, of course—I'm looking forward to *one of them* (you can guess which). And the other one I'll just have to be a good sport and try..."

As I scribbled down the recipes (given below) Julie continued, "She's going to serve the main courses with fresh pineapple and lots of flowers and Hawaiian music. Now, can you imagine wanting to eat *junk food* after this? No way!"

"Aloha!" I said, thinking, *and of course she's right.*

In the food department, *exciting* can be as important as healthy. I went away once again impressed by the energy and imagination of those Iowans!

Pickled Cucumber and Seaweed Salad
4 ounces wakame seaweed
1 cucumber, thinly sliced
½ cup white vinegar
2 tbsp. soy sauce
1 tbsp. shredded fresh ginger
1 tbsp. sugar
2 ounces minced clams
Serves six

1) Soak seaweed until tender (20 to 30 minutes).
2) Slice the cucumber, salt lightly, let stand 30 minutes. Drain liquid.
3) Cut the seaweed into 1-inch strips. Mix with vinegar, soy sauce, shredded ginger, and sugar.

4) Combine wakame, cucumber, and minced clams in a salad bowl. Pour in the vinegar-soy dressing, mix, and serve!

Kalua Roast Pig

(Maxine told me that in different parts of the world ti leaves, banana leaves, or palm leaves are used to wrap or cook food in because they keep in moisture and give flavor. For this recipe she bought dried palm leaves in the Oriental market in Dubuque. But of course, since she lives in Iowa, cornhusks are a good substitute!)

15 ti leaves or dried palm leaves, soaked to soften
5 pound pork picnic shoulder roast
2 tsp coarse salt
1½ tbsp. liquid smoke
¼ cup water

1) Preheat oven to 300°.
2) Line a deep roasting pan with ti leaves.
3) Salt the pork roast.
4) Cover meat with leaves and tie up with string.
5) Place wrapped meat in pan on top of leaves, then cover meat with more leaves.
6) Pour a mixture made of the liquid smoke and water over the meat and leaves.
7) Seal the pan tightly with aluminum foil to keep moisture in.
8) Roast the pork 3 hours or until very well done and to the point of overdone. The meat is taken off the bones and shredded by hand, never cut with a knife.

The Facts of Life

You wouldn't buy a car without knowing *something* about what you were buying, would you? Yet you make food choices every day, often without understanding the basics of what your body needs. You don't have to be a nutritionist to make good choices, but you have to know a few basic facts.

If your health is more important to you than your car, take the time to listen to Jane Clemen, Mercy nutritionist and Fight the Fat organizer. "Everyone's heard of the food pyramid, right? Well, it's not enough to know vaguely that it exists. The reason that the U.S. Department of Health came up with the image of a pyramid was so that a great deal of information could be packed into one powerful, easy-to-remember symbol. You should know it so well that when you close your eyes, you can *visualize* it. Make it a part of your life so that when you plan your meals, or when you shop for food, it is *always* there in the back of your mind. This way, making the right food choices will become second nature.

Note: Mayo Clinic has come up with a variation on the Food Pyramid that might work better since it allows you virtually unlimited vegetables and fruit and is geared toward weight loss (you can fill up on fruits and vegetables!). It is given below, as an alternative, after the traditional food pyramid.

The Food Pyramid

The Base: bread, cereals, rice, and pasta (6–11 servings).

Level Two: vegetables (3–5 servings) and fruits (2–4 servings).

Level Three: milk, yogurt, and cheese (2–3 servings), meat, poultry, fish, dry beans, eggs, and nuts (2–3 servings).

The Very Top of the Pyramid: fats and sweets. These are foods like salad dressings, cream, butter, margarine, sugars, soft drinks, candies, and sweet desserts. Alcoholic beverages are also part of this group. These foods provide calories but few vitamins and minerals.

What Is a Serving?
The Base
1 slice of bread

½ cup of cooked rice or pasta

½ cup of cooked cereal

1 ounce of ready-to-eat cereal

Level Two
Vegetables

½ cup chopped raw or cooked vegetables *minimum* (unlimited maximum)

1 cup of leafy raw vegetables *minimum* (unlimited maximum)

Fruit

1 piece of fruit or melon wedge

¾ cup of juice

½ cup of canned fruit

¼ cup of dried fruit

Level Three
1 cup of milk or yogurt

1½ ounces of natural cheese

2 ounces of processed cheese

2½ to 3 ounces of cooked, lean meat, poultry, or fish

Count ½ cup of cooked beans, 1 egg, or 2 tablespoons of peanut butter, and 1 ounce of lean meat.

The Very Top of the Pyramid
Limit calories from fats and sweets. To determine just how much leeway you have, see the chart on page 142.

How Many Servings Do You Need Each Day?

Food	Most Women	Children /Teenagers	Most Men
Bread Group	6	9	11
Vegetables	3	4	5
Fruits	2	3	4
Milk Group	2–3	2–3	2–3
Meat Group	2	2	3
Calories (approximate)	1,600	2,200	2,800

The Mayo Clinic Food Pyramid

The Base: the Mayo Clinic Food Pyramid has fruits and vegetables (both virtually unlimited) as the base or "first level." One serving of vegetables equals twenty-five calories, and one serving of fruit equals sixty calories. A serving size is two cups leafy vegetables, one cup vegetables, or one-half cup sliced fruit. You are required to eat a minimum of four servings of vegetables per day, three of fruit.

Level Two: in the Mayo Clinic Food Pyramid, bread, cereal, rice, and pasta are Level Two (four to eight servings per day). One serving equals one half-cup grain or cereal or one slice of bread, and is seventy calories.

Level Three: protein and dairy including beans, fish, lean meat, low-fat dairy (three to seven servings per day). One serving equals one-third cup beans, two to three ounces meat or fish, or one cup skim milk, and is seventy calories.

Level Four: olive oil, nuts, canola oil, and avocados (three to five servings per day) are healthy choices recommended.

Level Five: the tip of the pyramid includes candy and other sweets (up to 525 calories per week).

Note: physical activity is at the heart of the pyramid because of its central importance in weight management! See www.Mayo Clinic.com for other healthy suggestions.

The Rules of the Game
Calories

Calories measure the energy we get from food. They have often been compared to fuel—the fuel the body needs to keep going. A calorie measures energy in terms of heat, and it refers to the units of heat, or energy, which the body gets from its food. Heat given off by the fuel in a fireplace or furnace is measured in Thermal Units. Heat given off by the food in you is measured in calories. One calorie is the amount of energy needed to raise one gram of water one degree Celsius. Whether the calorie comes from carbohydrates, proteins, or fats, it represents the same amount of heat.

But what a difference it makes to you when you're trying to lose weight! Food is the fire that warms and invigorates you, the fuel that keeps you going in high gear. Yet one type of fuel burns low, sputters, smolders, and leaves a residue of ashes while another burns high and steady with a clean, bright flame. That's the way it is with the type of calories your body burns for energy. Think of food high in fat or loaded with processed sugar as the inefficient fuel billowing black smoke. And imagine the lean meats and low-fat dairy products, the veggies and fruits, filling your body with energy and strength!

Your *basal metabolism* represents the lowest number of calories required to maintain vital functions when you're sitting relaxed at a comfortable room temperature with your mind, body, and digestion completely at rest. Your metabolism starts to rise (above its basal level) about an hour after a meal, reaches its peak in about three hours, and by the sixth to eighth hour it drops back down to a fasting level. That's why you should never try to reduce by skipping meals. You can lose weight faster on the same amount of food if it's divided into several smaller meals throughout the day, as reformed breakfast skippers can testify.

Stoking up the Fires!

According to Jane Clemen, Dyersville Mercy Medical Center Director of Nutrition, of all foods, protein causes the most sustained rise in metabolism. Carbohydrates cause the least. The person who gains weight easily and seems unable to lose even on an extremely low-calorie diet may be one of the many whose body fails to burn up its carbohydrate calories at a normal rate. When not utilized, these calories pile up quickly as fat.

When your input and output are equal your weight remains normal, but take in more food than you burn and you will gain. Take in less food than you burn and you create a calorie deficit that causes a weight loss. Each pound of fat on your body represents thirty-five hundred calories. *To lose a pound requires a deficit of thirty-five hundred calories.* Cut your calorie intake by thirty-five hundred calories over a given time and within that time you will lose a pound.

The principle itself is sound, and you can lose weight at the specified rate, but do you have the willpower to cut your daily calorie intake by one third? Or to slash seven thousand calories out of your weekly meals for the sake of losing two pounds?

Type of calories can be as important as number! A low-calorie diet that doesn't have enough protein to raise the metabolism and burn stored fat slows weight loss and leaves you feeling half starved. Sufficient protein eases your hunger pangs and sustains your metabolism so that burning of fat for energy occurs. Bottom line: you lose weight faster than you did on fewer calories. Which makes the following information particularly useful: sixty to seventy-five grams of protein per day is an appropriate amount in a weight-loss diet. For example, six ounces of meat equals forty-two grams. Sixteen ounces of milk or yogurt equals sixteen grams. You can see how these are adding up. With so much conflicting advice, what can a dieter believe? Well, the following is *for sure*: unsaturated vegetable oils (such as safflower oil) are essential for your health, and when used in moderation can actually help you lose weight. Restrict the saturated fats by trimming the fat from your meat and being careful with your gravies and sauces and being especially cautious when it comes to butter and whole milk (either switch to margarine and skim milk or measure the amounts you use).

Weight loss depends both on what you eat and your portion sizes. Low-carbohydrate fruits and vegetables supply the energy value in a meal. You can get fat while eating small amounts of one type of food, and grow thin while eating large meals of another. When you know which foods should form the basis of your meals and which ones should be restricted or omitted, you can lose weight without going hungry.

Now go back and check out the food pyramid on page 140. When you can close your eyes and visualize it right away, from the grains on the bottom to the fats and sugars on the top, you'll know you've studied it the way you should have!

The Basic Math of Weight Loss

The bottom line for determining daily caloric totals is the following formula: the calories an individual needs to *maintain* his or her weight = ten times their weight.

Example: Vivian weighs 200 pounds.
200 x 10 = 2,000 calories per day

To lose one pound, you must consume thirty-five hundred calories less than you need, or exercise to burn those calories. So, if Vivian consumes fifteen hundred calories every day instead of the two thousand she needs for maintenance, by the end of the week she'll be down thirty-five hundred calories, or one pound.

Of course, all kinds of variables can kick in. She might be holding water and when she loses that pound, she'll lose another "bonus" pound from cutting her salt intake. Or, she might be doing a lot of exercising and revving up her metabolism—the payoff can then be another bonus pound gone. But the basic principle of weight loss works this way: once you have taken in thirty-five hundred fewer calories than you need to maintain your weight, you will lose a pound. Five minutes of attention to the math chart equals a thinner, healthier you! If you can multiply and add, then you can do the mathematics of weight loss—if you can't, buy a calculator!

If you're lazy, you can check in with www.ediets.com, a great new option offered at a discount to members of last year's Fight the Fat. You punch in such information as your weight, height, age, etc., and they set up individual meal plans together with individual workouts and recipes. It's like getting an accountant to handle your money. But even if you get them to help start you off, there's a huge advantage to knowing what you're doing. The knowledge will come in handy in all kinds of day-to-day situations your computer can't figure out in advance for you.

There's no substitute for putting your mind to healthy menus and figuring out what's right for you by way of nutrition. Studying the basic facts of nutrition forces you to *focus*. And being successful at weight loss is like success at tennis or golf: it's a matter of attention, and of concentration. By putting some time and care into improving your health and eating habits, you are making a commitment. The person who's given serious thought to preparing a healthy, well-balanced dinner *won't be as likely* to throw away that time and effort at the sound of the ice cream truck! Make sure you know if you have enough calories in the bank before you spend those calories!

A Short Survey of the Basic Principles of Nutrition

The three keys to good nutrition: balance! Balance! Balance! Carbohydrates, proteins, and fats all have important functions. The American Heart Association, the National Cholesterol Education Program, and the American Cancer Society recommend that 10 to 15 percent of calories come from protein, fifty-five to sixty from carbohydrates, and no more than 30 percent from fat.

Carbohydrates are the important source of energy glucose for our bodies. If we don't consume enough carbohydrates, the body breaks down lean body mass and then fat in an effort to provide glucose to the central nervous system. Protein is important for normal growth and maintaining lean muscle mass. It is also important in the repair of body tissue after an injury or surgery. Protein in the absence of carbohydrates (glucose) will be converted to glucose and used as an energy source.

Fat provides our bodies with essential fatty acids, helps with normal body function, and is used by the body for energy (that's why *some* fat, a limited amount, is necessary). But keep in mind: 1 gram fat = 9 calories, 1 gram of protein or carbohydrate = 4 calories, and 1 gram of alcohol = 7 calories.

The American Heart Association recommends that no more than 30 percent of total calories eaten in one day come from fat—an important strategy in reducing your risk of heart disease.

The absence of any of these important nutrients affects the utilization of the others and may put you at increased risk for problems down the road. The best nutritional guide for providing variety and balance is the Food Guide Pyramid. Each of the five major food groups provides essential nutrients.

Bread, cereal, rice, and pasta provide carbohydrates for energy, B vitamins, thiamin, niacin, iron, and fiber. Vegetables provide significant amounts of a variety of vitamins and minerals. You need to include a good source of vitamin A and beta-carotene at least every other day—dark green, leafy vegetables and orange vegetables. Fruits also provide large amounts of vitamins and minerals and include a good source of vitamin C daily. Choose skim or low-fat milk; dairy is the most important source of calcium and is a very good source of protein and riboflavin, a B vitamin. Meat, poultry, fish, dry beans, eggs, and nuts provide significant amounts of protein and iron, niacin and thiamin.

Omitting any of these food groups could result in deficiencies of one or more major nutrients. This is not a problem for short periods of time, but it is a nutritional disaster of the first order when followed for more than two weeks. The recommended number of servings depends on your stage of life and how active you are. For weight loss, most of us should stay at the low end of ranges for each food group.

Fats, sweets, and oils provide calories, but few vitamins and minerals. Keep these to a minimum! They don't give you anything but *weight*!

Menus from the Dyersville Restaurants

Many Dyersville restaurants participated in Fight the Fat: the Cardinal Lounge, LeRoy's Pizza & Restaurant, the Ritz Restaurant, Dyersville McDonald's, Dyersville Subway, the Country Junction Restaurant. In addition, the local supermarket, Payless, not only acted as one of the sponsors, but they also cooperated by putting up signs indicating which were the best food choices according to Fight the Fat.

The restaurateurs worked out the nutritional and caloric values and the fat content of their food with Mercy nutritionist Jane Clemen. The menus they produced are an example of what can be done when a team of determined people decides to make a difference.

The owner of Dyersville's Cardinal Lounge joined Fight the Fat and did very well on the program. During the first Fight the Fat she hosted a pre-meeting dinner that featured a lean beef roll up course, a salad bar adapted to Fight the Fat advice and a low-calorie version of peach cobbler. She noticed that during and after the campaign, her customers ordered differently—mainly from the special Fight the Fat menus. "Of course there are still customers who want an extra large steak and a double order of potatoes, but during and after the campaign, we sold more and more healthy food. And it's a pattern that has continued. Fight the Fat has been great for the community."

The managers of the Country Junction Restaurant have also gone out of their way to offer special lean lunches and have added entrées that are appetizing without adding loads of calories to the meal. It's a popular restaurant and reports a good response to the low-fat cuisine: another example of the law of supply-and-demand working in favor of healthy choices.

To give you an idea of Fight the Fat's eating out possibilities, here are menus from the Ritz, LeRoy's Pizza, and Dyersville's McDonald's.

The Ritz Restaurant

According to Jeff Ehlers, owner and a strong supporter of Fight the Fat, "The Heart Smart logo next to an item means seven grams of fat or less. Ostrich and Cajun chicken breast are two examples. Ostrich tastes like tenderloin, some say like beef fillet mignon. We raise them locally, about twenty miles from here on my brother-in-law's farm. The Ritz shrimp or the scallops are a good choice, as long as you get them broiled, not deep fried. Teams come in frequently during the campaign, and sometimes you'll get couples with one of them eating heart smart and the other not. We try to cater to everyone!"

Ritz Restaurant Menu

Suggested low*er* fat items from the menu:
Broiled Cod (210 Calories, 1.7 grams fat)
Cajun Chicken Breast (375 calories, 8 grams fat)
Broiled Orange Roughy (200 calories, 2 grams fat)
Broiled Shrimp (140 calories, 1.5. grams fat)
Broiled Scallops (190 calories, 5.6 grams fat)
Cajun Pork Loin (290 calories, 11.5 grams fat)
Broiled Seafood Platter (250 calories, 4.3 grams fat)
Ritz Shrimp (150 calories, 2.4 grams fat)
Ostrich Meat, 5 oz. (142 calories, 3 grams fat)
Open-faced Beef Tenderloin Sandwich (370 calories, 12.3 grams fat)
Boneless Chicken Breast/Kaiser Roll (310 calories, 6.3 grams fat)
Seven-Inch Vegetable Pizza (365 calories, 12.3 grams fat)
Suggested Accompaniments: Baked Potato, Tossed Salad with Low-Fat Dressing, Dinner Roll

LeRoy's Pizza & Restaurant

Duanne Ott, owner and a strong supporter of Fight the Fat, says, "My pizza is low-fat. As a result of Fight the Fat, we measured ingredients more carefully. We made a list of certain items and did calorie counts on them. The nutritionist from one of our suppliers and the nutritionist from the Dyersville Mercy Medical Center helped us make sure we were 100 percent accurate.

"This year, Tuesday night is meeting night and afterwards we had lots of teams come in for low-fat pizza and salads. We have made pizza a diet food with vegetables and skim mozzarella and being careful about exactly how much cheese we put on it. We have plans for a whole wheat pizza and an all-veggie, no-cheese pizza as well.

"Over the last years I've seen patterns in town change a lot. You see many more people ordering the grilled chicken breast. When they order cod, they get it steamed rather than fried. They ask for baked potatoes. Because there's been so much concern about fat, we've made sure to have low-calorie, low-fat salad dressing on supply—more people ask for it than any other dressing. Overall, people here have been going toward healthier eating. They start out during the ten weeks and then continue to change over the whole year."

LeRoy's Pizza & Restaurant Menu

Suggested low*er* fat items from the menu:
Mini Vegetable Pizza (230 calories, 8.2 grams fat)
Mini Meatless Taco Pizza (285 calories, 9.2 grams fat)
Large Seafood Salad w/No-Fat Ranch Dressing
(310 calories, 7 grams fat)
Grilled Chicken Breast Salad w/No-Fat Ranch Dressing
(260 calories, 5 grams fat—request without cheese or egg yolk)
Grilled Chicken Breast Sandwich (360 calories, 7.3 grams fat)
Low-Fat Chili (250 calories, 8.5 grams fat)

Dyersville's McDonald's

Jennifer, the manager, worked out this menu for Fight the Fat members. She wanted to make sure that they could still eat at McDonald's and stay on the Fight the Fat low-fat plan:

Meal #1
1 Hamburger
1 Side Salad
No-fat Herb Dressing
355 calories, 9 grams fat

Meal #2
1 Bowl Chicken Noodle Soup
1 Garden Salad
No-fat Herb Dressing
205 calories, 2 grams fat

Meal #3
1 Grilled Chicken, No Mayonnaise
1 Side Salad
No-fat Herb Dressing
225 calories, 3 grams fat

Meal #4
1 Bowl Vegetable Beef Soup
1 Garden Salad
No-fat Herb Dressing
335 calories, 11 grams fat

Meal #5
1 Bowl of Cream Potato Soup
1 Garden Salad
No-fat Herb Dressing
420 calories, 7 grams fat

Meal #6
1 Grilled Chicken, No Mayonnaise
1 Bowl of Chicken Soup
305 calories, 10 grams fat

Meal #7
1 Grilled Chicken, No Mayonnaise
1 Bowl of Vegetable Beef Soup
440 calories, 8 grams fat

Meal #8
1 Chicken Fajita
1 Garden Salad
No-fat Herb Dressing
275 calories, 7 grams fat

Substitutions or Add-Ons
1 Grilled Chicken Salad =120 calories and 1.5 grams fat
Reduced French Dressing =160 calories and 8 grams fat
Light Mayonnaise = 40 calories and 4 grams fat

Desserts
Reduced-Fat Vanilla Ice Cream Cone =150 calories and 4.5 grams fat
Strawberry Sundae = 290 calories and 7 grams fat
1 Package McDonald-Land Cookies =180 calories and 5 grams fat

Beverages
1% Low-fat Milk =100 calories and 2.5 grams fat
Orange Juice = 80 calories and 0 grams fat

Breakfast Entrées
Low-fat Apple Bran Muffin = 300 calories and 3 grams fat
1 Order of Plain Hotcakes and 1 Package of Jelly = 375 calories and 8 grams fat
1 English Muffin and 1 Package of Jelly=190 calories and 2 grams fat
1 Hash Brown = 305 calories and 10 grams fat
2 Eggs, Scrambled =160 calories and 11 grams fat
1 Plain Bagel = 250 calories and 1 gram fat

Extras
Jelly = 35 calories and 0 grams fat
Light Cream Cheese = 60 calories and 4.5 grams fat

Fight the Fat Shopping List

Payless Foods, the Dyersville Supermarket, helped out by tagging products recommended for Fight the Fat members with small yellow laminated signs saying *Fight the Fat Wise Choice.* Walking down the aisles, Fight the Fat members found it a cinch to shop here.

This is a sampling of recommended products:

Fat-free cheese	Egg Beaters
Tuna in water	English Muffins
Pickles	Melba snacks
Snackwell crackers	Fat-free cottage cheese
Fat-free lunch meat	Nonfat sour cream
Fat-free ranch, western dressing	Low-fat or nonfat yogurt
Dubuque extra-lean ham and turkey	V8 juice
Chef's choice, stir-fry	Pasta
Premium ground beef	Juice
Turkey breast	Light pancake syrup
Chicken breast	Regular popcorn
Reduced-fat peanut butter	Fat-free Pringles
Reduced-fat Triscuits	Snack pack Jell-O
Skim milk	

Supermarkets anywhere can attract business by inviting a dietician to identify wise choices, labeling them, and promoting them.

Your Workbook

Exercises, Questions, Tips, & Points to Ponder for Week 7 of Fight the Fat

The Bulletin Board

"Many [people] have a wrong idea of what constitutes true happiness. It is not attained through self-gratification, but through faithfulness to a worthy goal."
—Hellen Keller

"Discovery consists of looking at the same thing as everyone else and thinking something different."
—Albert Szent-Gyorgyi

"I've been through every diet under the sun, and I can tell you that getting up and getting out and walking is always the first goal."
—Oprah Winfrey

"If you rest, you rust!"
—Helen Hayes

Eleanor Roosevelt grew up surrounded by great wealth and great sadness. She lost her mother who showed little love for Eleanor when she was eight and her father, who truly loved her, when she was nine. Later in life, she made great discoveries within herself of intelligence, compassion, strength, and a true understanding of wealth. When Eleanor died, Adlai Stevenson said of her, "She would rather light candles than curse the darkness."

"You must do the thing you think you cannot do!"
—Eleanor Roosevelt

"No one can make you feel inferior without your consent."
—Eleanor Roosevelt

"The body is a sacred garment."
—Martha Graham

Your Journal

Every time you look at a billboard or a magazine, models are sending you a message. As a culture, we are obsessed with certain looks as opposed to certain healthy goals.

When you are surrounded by these super-thin images and bombarded by these "get gaunt" messages, it takes self-knowledge to resist. It takes thoughtfulness to make a healthy counterstatement. It takes sanity and wisdom to ignore the hype and pressure from the vanity industries. Use your journal to respond. Write up a declaration of independence! Explore the ways in which your goals differ from those advocating the anorexic look!

Healthy Habit for the Week

Don't forget to figure in the fiber factor when making up your menu. Not only does it keep digestion running smoothly, but research has also shown that foods containing fiber can lower blood cholesterol, improve blood sugar levels, facilitate the absorption of nutrients, *and* protect against cancer.

Sources: whole grains, nuts, seeds, fruits, and vegetables. To be considered a good source of fiber, a cereal should give you at least four grams of bran per one-ounce serving. Cooked beans are an excellent source—especially pinto, navy, and kidney beans—whole grains, vegetables, and fruits are also good fiber foods. Besides providing fiber, prunes are also a good source of vitamin A and potassium, are nonfat, and have no cholesterol and sodium!

Apart from the nutritional reasons, there's a good physiological reason to eat fiber too: fiber foods make you feel full and add to your well-being.

Reward for the Week

Get away from it all while staying at home. Of course it's great to get out and see a play, go to a movie, a comedy club, a concert, or a ballet. You can't always do this, but you can create a *night at the movies* at *home* by making certain simple rules: turn off the phone and turn down the answering machine. Make your movie time *your* time (already, from establishing your exercise time, your long hot bath time, and your night out at Fight the Fat meetings, your family has come to understand the concept of sacred time! Time when you can't be interrupted. No requests from them are honored during these times. And anything short of the house being on fire *can wait*).

Try a new movie, or, even better, rent an old one that you loved and haven't seen for years. Forgetting everyone and everything for two hours is just what the doctor ordered. A tear-jerker, a thigh-slapper, suit yourself, just make sure you *are* suiting yourself and not watching along as your spouse enjoys him/herself. This one is *for you*—for having completed another week on program.

Team Activity for the Week

Together with your teammates, branch out into something totally new. There are hundreds of examples, from taking classes in pottery (very stimulating *and* soothing at the same time) or fencing (a wonderful outlet for aggression and as demanding as dance) to horseback riding (a form of exercise that will add so much zest to your life and is available to you even in the largest cities). *Pottery or painting classes!* Who has time for this you ask? The answer is: *you do!* You have an incredible amount of time—use it properly! Use it for things that will enrich your life and things that you can turn to in moments of stress.

An ideal possibility for this activity is overnight hiking. This suggestion is a particularly good one since it combines many elements that Fight the Fat has been emphasizing: breaking out of old routines, using nature as a source of inspiration, getting more motion into your life. If you've been working on your walking or running it'll be easier to lose yourself in nature—the physical part of the hike will be demanding, but you'll be prepared for it. You and your teammate(s) can determine the level of the hike.

In any case, knowing that the hike is coming up is a wonderful way of keeping your eye on a tangible goal. *I want to be able to enjoy that hike, so I better not skip my aerobics class tonight!* Awakening in the woods is an awesome experience. And the break in your routine is a huge stress reliever. All your senses are heightened by the unusual experience, and the wild flowers or streams or mossy rocks that you chance upon as you wander will make you forget that you are burning up calories.

For details about how to organize an overnight in the woods, you can call a hiking club near you, or you can call the Sierra Club at (415) 977-5653, or the American Hiking Society at (301) 565-6704 ext. 605. Stores like Eastern Mountain Sports and Recreational Equipment, Inc. (REI) also run free clinics.

Golden Rule for the Week

Repetition helps. Call it focus, paying attention, becoming conscious, auto-suggestion—even call it brainwashing!—who cares what name you give it as long as it works, right?

Repeat slogans, inspirational sayings, and helpful rules until they become a part of you. Go over them again and again in the car on the way to work, in the shower, or on your walk. They will become like a mantra and in times of temptation, these auto-suggestions will save you: *nothing is as good as thin tastes! There's nothing that one bite won't make worse! Willpower is like a muscle—the more you use it, the stronger it becomes!*

How many childhood poems or rules do we think of because we had to memorize them? How powerful a tool is repetition in music or in poetry!

It is the same principle here: what you repeat or memorize becomes a part of you. And what is a part of you becomes a reflex, an automatic response in times of stress.

Food of the Week

Did you know that *spinach*:
1) Revs up the metabolism?
2) Is a natural laxative?
3) Provides large doses of calcium, iron, and vitamin A?
4) Is rich in beta-carotene, vitamins C and E, and other nutrients?
5) Is a protector against cancer?
6) Lowers cholesterol?

Spinach does all that according to the *Journal of American Medicine*, and requires no more than a minute or two steaming or stir-frying to prepare.

Low-fat (or Fat-free) Dairy! An excellent source of protein—just be sure that it really is low-fat. Check out the percentages and calories from fat when you buy it.

Garlic. A raw clove or two of garlic (a clove is one of the sections of the bulb) is good for more than just keeping vampires away. Some studies state that this pungent pleaser may prevent blood clots, reduce the risk of stroke and heart disease, and lower the cholesterol levels by as much as 10 percent. It is an antiviral that also fights twelve different strains of bacteria, some resistant to antibiotics (during WWII soldiers used garlic when they ran out of penicillin), which is why it's good for people with chronic infections.

Garlic-consuming cultures have far fewer cases of stomach and colon cancer. Garlic's virtues are almost unbelievable—yet there are people who just can't stand its odor (I'll bet they haven't even read to the bottom of this paragraph). And of course, there are garlic lovers for whom it's next door to a perfume. Some say that if you eat it regularly and chew a little parsley afterwards, you'll be okay in that respect. The beneficial health effects of garlic are most powerful when the garlic is eaten raw (or added in the last stages of cooking).

Self-empowerment Exercise for the Week

"Laughter is inner jogging."
—Norman Cousins

"If you're going to be able to look back on something and laugh about it, you might as well laugh about it now."
—Marie Osmond

"If you choose one characteristic that [will] get you through life, choose a sense of humor!"
—Jennifer Jones

"If you can laugh at it, you can live with it!"
—Erma Bombeck

Stress, tension, worry, pain—they all dissolve in laughter. Weight loss is a serious business. It affects your health, your energy level, your appearance, and your ability to have a well-rounded, full life. But acknowledging its seriousness doesn't mean you can't have some fun getting rid of those excess pounds. And that's what Fight the Fat is all about: goofy gags, jokes, stories, swapping anecdotes about successes and failures. Learning how to laugh at yourself, to see yourself through the eyes of others, and to share your experiences with people who are striving towards the same goal.

Laughter is a kind of alchemy, only instead of changing base metals to gold it changes pain to joy.

Rosalie Kaufman, author of *Yes You Can!,* begins her account of her fifty-pound weight loss this way: "I had only one goal: it wasn't to write the great American novel, it wasn't to be First Lady—it was to get out of my maternity clothes...and I wasn't even pregnant!" The ability to have a good laugh at yourself is freeing, and liberating.

One member decided to see all the old Chaplin classics and laughed her way into a state of euphoria. Actually, all those belly laughs produce a physiological result as well as a psychological one. When you laugh hard, you take in more oxygen and provide the body with a much needed release of tension. *Always* laugh when you can. It's cheap medicine.

So, start laughing! There is so much comic material available—tapes, books, videos, plays. George Burns's memoirs are bestsellers, for example, because people love the humorous way he describes his life. He puts his readers into a good mood instantly; he makes it possible for them to go back to their own life situations with a lighter heart. Swap jokes with your teammates. Try to see everything from the point of view of an angel, since, as the saying goes, *Angels fly because they take themselves so lightly.*

Stress Antidote for the Week

"Music! The moody food of us who deal in love!"
Shakespeare's *Antony and Cleopatra*

A great escape when you feel stressed out and unhappy and are on the verge of going for the ice cream and cookies is *music*. Don't just stick to what you know—branch out! Experiment with different kinds from Country Western to Gregorian Chant; you never know what you will come across that will do the trick. The popularity of Gregorian Chant was probably a result of the fact that so many people felt calmer after listening to the low, soothing sounds of the monks' voices. I remember hearing them from the convertible of a red Ferrari stuck next to me in an L.A. freeway traffic jam! They really took you out of the stressful moment and brought you to where you wanted to be!

A physiological change actually occurs when you listen to music. It can soothe you and leave you feeling ready to face the world—without that candy bar or hot fudge sundae. In addition to solitary listening, your team can go out *together* to a musical event. It's so much more fun to attend a concert when you're with friends. Members can swap CDs and listening suggestions at meetings or even begin meetings with the playing of some special work. Music is also a great motivator for exercise. It's easier to keep going while "holding on to" some song that's running through your head.

While not everybody is gifted, everybody can enjoy the fun of playing an instrument—a powerful *replacement* for food. Instead of opening up the fridge, sit down at the piano or pick up the guitar.

Fight the Fat member Joyce of Dyersville, a member of the Dyersville Hardee's team, the *Starlites*, shares her gifts with others as well as benefiting from them herself. "I had a guitar group that played in church. We were three players and one or two singers, and we really loved making music together. Now we play in the nursing home once or twice a month on Sundays and recently we've been asked to play for birthday parties or other special events…we give whatever money we make to charity."

Chapter Eight: Look Out, World

"It is not the mountain we conquer, but ourselves."
—Sir Edmund Hillary, famed New Zealand mountain climber,
known for his conquest of Mount Everest

"Success is a journey, not a destination.
The doing is usually more important than the outcome."
—Arthur Ashe

Why will this time be different from all the other times? *You have a buddy or a team to support you.* So? *So!* Nobody can be inspired, motivated, and revved up *all the time.* That's where your buddy comes in. It doesn't matter whether you're a duo or part of a five–hundred–member convention—a small spark starts a large flame. When you're feeling down, you can now turn to another person who is working alongside you. She's not a professional counselor—they have their own function and they can be useful in their own way—but this is different. Your buddy or your teammate is not being paid to help you. She's someone who is struggling as hard as you are, who's making mistakes and working to correct them, who's learning about food, who's exercising, and trying to chill out with every antistress technique she can! She probably loves ice cream as much as you do—and hates broccoli more! Her successes are yours and yours are hers. That's the discovery of Fight the Fat.

Marlene, a waitress in a Dyersville restaurant popular among Fight the Fat members, says, "Sometimes you don't want to talk to your family about something, even when you're close. You want to talk to someone who's going through the same thing you are. The teams come in here to eat after exercising, and I see what goes on. They linger. They talk. They tell each other they can do it."

But what is that spark called motivation? It comes and goes, sometimes for no reason you can figure out. It's a feeling, a mood, something that seems unreal or intangible, yet it's the most important part of the Fight the Fat campaign, and translates into very tangible, very real results. With it, you can do anything. You can put up with anything; you can fail a hundred times and still end up succeeding. Without it, nothing is possible, the smallest obstacle becomes a mountain.

When I asked Dyersville *Hips Hips Away* team member Viv to define motivation, she said: "I can't define it. But I know it when I feel it." Fair enough. So let's try an experiment. Read the following quotes one after the other without interruption:

"Everybody wants to be Cary Grant. Even I want to be Cary Grant."
—Cary Grant

"Courage is nothing less than the power to overcome danger, misfortune, fear, injustice, while continuing to affirm inwardly that life with all its sorrows is good; that everything is meaningful even if in a sense beyond our understanding; and that there is always tomorrow."
—Dorothy Thompson

"I do not try to dance better than anyone else.
I only try to dance better than myself."
—Mikhail Baryshnikov

"Weight lifting is all 'mind over matter.' As long as the mind can envision the fact that you can do something, you can. I visualize myself being there already—having achieved the goal already. Working out is just the physical follow through, a reminder of the vision you're focusing on."
—Arnold Schwarzenegger

"The wise man in the storm prays to God not for safety from danger, but for deliverance from fear. It is the storm within that endangers him."
—Ralph Waldo Emerson

"Don't tell me I can't do something. Don't tell me it's impossible.
Don't tell me I'm not the greatest. I'm the double greatest."
—Muhammad Ali

"Shoot for the moon. If you miss, you land among the stars."
—Les Brown

"Life is what you make it...always has been, always will be."
—Grandma Moses

"A problem faced up to, is a problem half solved."
—Professor Maura Spiegal, Columbia University

"Strength does not come from winning. Your struggles develop your strengths.
When you go through hardships and decide not to surrender, that is strength."
—Arnold Schwarzenegger

"It does not matter how slowly you go so long as you do not stop."
—Confucius

"Good people are good because they've come to wisdom through failure.
We get very little wisdom from success, you know."
—William Saroyan

"Last week I saw a woman who had not made a mistake in 3,000 years.
She was a mummy in the Metropolitan Museum."
—Christiane Menzel

"If we learn from the experience, there is no failure—only delayed victory."
—Carrie Chapman Catt

"Old age is not so bad when you consider the alternatives."
—Maurice Chevalier, actor

Don't you feel as if you have stood in the sun for a few moments or taken a sip of wine? You just got a double dose of the vitamin *I Can* with some *laughter* mixed in! Consider how you felt before and how you feel now. In just a few minutes, after listening to voices that were inspired, that had joy in them, wisdom in them, and strength in them, you've caught some of that inspiration, joy, wisdom, and strength. That's the way motivation works. And that's why any team, whether it has two members or two hundred, should put aside time to discuss inspirational books, quotes, and tapes. Invite speakers when possible and view their videos when it's not. It's as simple, and as crucial, as that.

Listening to these kinds of "strengthening" thoughts deepens your commitment, strengthens your resolve, and makes you want to keep going. A steady diet of negative thoughts, pessimism, defeatism, and self-criticism can keep you stuck in the mud. "It'll never last! I'm not a joiner! (from a woman whose weight is causing serious problems when she tries walking). I know I could do it if I started—but I just can't start!" These are common remarks made by people hopelessly addicted to sugar and sweets and weighed down not by pounds but by their thoughts! A steady *diet* of inspiration can raise your spirits and make each day better than the one before. What you chose to listen to is up to you.

Once you are motivated, though, the real challenge is to stay that way. The best rule for this sounds like a catch-22. If you want to *remain* motivated *realize it won't last!* Or, as Zig Zigler put it, "People often say that motivation doesn't last. Well, neither does bathing! That's why we recommend it daily!"

By joining Fight the Fat, you are planning in advance for those times when you feel *I can't, I just can't.* That's why many of the teams keep working together after the formal ten weeks of Fight the Fat are over. I met with one such team at the end of the fourth Fight the Fat. The "captain," Julie, had been a member of Dyersville's *Phil's Fannies* last year (that's a team made up of nine elementary school teachers whose principal was Phil!). After the ten-week campaign was over, she felt that she was "just getting started," so she teamed up with a buddy. "My other teammates lived a distance," she told me, "and I wanted to have frequent meetings. That's why I made up a mini-team with my friend Mary—we call it *Two Against the World* since it's just the two of us."

"I'd been in two Fight the Fats," her buddy Mary added, "though never on Julie's team (I was a member of *Never Again-2-Fat*. We're a Dyersville-based team of seven good friends). And I noticed how hard things got for me inbetween. So, I walked down the block and knocked on Julie's door—I really had to laugh because she said she was planning to come to me the next day. We just decided to keep on going from where we'd left off at the end of the campaign."

"I really needed it," Julie said. "It keeps me in line if I know I'll be seeing Mary over the weekend, or that we'll be meeting together after work. If I've made an appointment to go power walking with Mary, there's no way I'll break it. After all, it's even more important now since she's my whole team! And if I put in an hour walking, there's no way I'm going to pig out afterward."

"Please! I don't like that expression," says her buddy. "I've been telling Julie that I think it takes away from our dignity to talk that way! We have to work on our self-esteem."

"You can see we're a perfect team," laughed Julie. "We disagree all the time! That's why we take turns being "captain"—next week she's it."

"How do you keep up your motivation?" I asked.

"The first thing is, we exercise together," Julie answered. "That's very important for both of us."

"Sometimes we'll cook a big *healthy* dinner for both our families," Mary said. "Either I'll come over here or she'll come to my place and we'll work together. It's a lot of fun—we'll make some secret treats and the kids have to guess what's in it. Half the time, they can't!"

"Another thing," Julie put in. "We'll go shopping together. You'd be surprised how important it is to get support at the mall. We have young kids and when we took them to the mall in Dubuque, we really used to get in trouble."

"The kids drag you into the food court for lunch," Mary groaned. "Many things on the menu are super-fat. Just one slice of pepperoni pizza can be as much as five hundred calories and twenty-one grams of fat. And ten of those grams can be saturated."

"I used to have one or two slices of spinach & broccoli stuffed pizza when I visited my relatives out of state," Julie said indignantly, "and I thought I was really being good. But it turned out that what I was eating had as much fat as the pepperoni and gave me seven hundred calories. Not to mention the baked ziti and meat lasagna at seven hundred to eight hundred calories! *Nutrition Action* even said that when they tested the so-called "diet" veggie pizza they'd ordered at various pizza parlors, many times they were served the regular vegetable pizza instead—six hundred and fifty calories isn't low-calorie. No wonder I kept putting on weight."

Mary nodded and added, "So, I keep *her* out of trouble, and she keeps me away from double fudge brownies and its—"

"Wait a minute," Julie interrupted. "Let's not *dwell* on the brownies and the etceteras—what's the point? If you really want something from there, have it, don't dream about it!"

"I don't need to this week!" Mary shook her head.

"Okay, then let's think about the tuna casserole and cheesy hash browns. We can have that made Fight the Fat–style for half the calories. You see, " Julie turned to me with a smile, "this is what we go through when the mall comes up."

"Well," I said, "I wouldn't want to be eating brownies in the mall *this month*." And we all laughed because we were picturing the same scene: the food court at Kennedy Mall in Dubuque where *this year* unhealthy food was definitely *out*. Sbarro's on one side, the Great American Cookie Factory on the other, two hundred and fifty overweight people in the middle exercising—they were trying out every kind of activity under the sun from jazzercize to cardio-karate. Every ten minutes, a whistle was blown and the teams switched to different trainers! For a "cool off" the team members wandered among the various restaurants that had put up table tents listing nutritional values and fat content!

If this sounds like a dream, try coming down to the mall on a Monday night. That's where the Dubuque Fight the Fat is being held. "We were looking for a place with a sound system and plenty of room for people to exercise," said Fight the Fat organizer Dianna Kirkwood, an organizer behind the Dubuque event. "It was just a question of getting a dietitian to talk to the various restaurateurs, to find out whether there was anything suitable for us on their menus. And they were very cooperative—we uncovered some possibilities, and they listed the information to help our members make good choices. The people running the mall were delighted to give us the space for free—it brought in customers. Specifically, five hundred of them. We had to run the meeting in two shifts, 5 PM and 7 PM! So, Monday night at the mall means *fitness* now!"

This huge event provides a perfect addition to Julie and Mary's miniteam. These two women strolling with their kids in the mall, helping each other make the right choices, are just as much in the spirit of Fight the Fat as the big team event. The idea is the same: develop healthy patterns that can be sustained; try out new things; tap into the strength and energy that comes from offering support to others and receiving it in turn.

There's support all around you *if you chose to tap into it.* The bottom line is that you know where you can turn when you're feeling down. You know instinctively who will support you and who will try to drag you back toward your old habits. It's a question of which way you *really* want to go.

Secret Teammates

One way to get with it is to find your "secret teammate." The sources of support are sometimes not official ones. It could be that the someone who brightens your day, and makes you feel good about yourself or about the way you look is your "secret" teammate. For example, the Dyersville Subway restaurant kept coming up again and again as I spoke to various members from different teams. They would start out by talking about what they could have for lunch or dinner there and still be eating on a low-fat, healthy food plan. But more often than not, the manager Brenda was just as important an attraction as the food.

Curious to see what was going on, I visited Subway and talked to Brenda, who presented an interesting angle on how Fight the Fat works, even though at the time she herself had not yet joined.

An attractive, vital person, Brenda had been influenced by the Fight the Fat teams coming into Subway after meetings. The program inspired her to think up ways to help others. The tips she gave them and her attitude made all the difference—and finally all that support she gave others ended up strengthening her as well. This year she is a member of the program and is a great example of the Fight the Fat philosophy.

"Jane Clemen is a friend of the family," Brenda started to explain how it started during her break, while still keeping an eye on the counter. For her, working at Subway is something she *enjoys*. She's a people person who really cares about her customers, as I was to see by the way that they greeted her and the advice she gave them.

"So, when Jane proposed that our Subway join the campaign," she went on, "I was really excited. Even before that, I've been trying to watch what I eat. And I'm lucky working at Subway since as long as I watch my cheese and mayo, I can do well eating here."

"In terms of calories?"

"Calories, fats—Subway food can be very healthy."

"What do you have on the menu especially for Fight the Fat?" I asked.

"Well, first of all, when Fight the Fat members come in and start ordering, we usually give them a nutritional guide to Subway (we also give it out at the meetings). I omit the cheese, for starters. I always say, 'Are you part of the Fight the Fat program? Because if you are, I can help you out. You won't miss the cheese, and if you shy away from the mayo and want a little more flavor, put on a little mustard and use the vinegar and spices…oregano works quite well.' It's a question of being smart about what you eat.

"I try to show them what's possible here. If you really want to cheat, just a little, I can help you out with that too. I mean, we can fix up something that's not really bad for you—they can cheat without going overboard.

"And they love it. They come in here and ask, 'Well, how many grams of fat does this have? Am I under my limit?' And I'm, 'Oh yeah! You can have that.' I have regular customers I serve all the time, and you see a lot of changes in the way they've been eating because of Fight the Fat. There are a couple of individuals especially who have made massive changes over three years. If you look at them from the beginning till now, they've really done well at keeping it off. They've changed their whole eating habits. One girl comes in at least twice a week and she's amazing. She looks like a completely different person. So much better."

"Do you compliment her on it?"

"Oh, definitely, I'm always saying to her, 'You are looking great.' And she told me, 'You never realize that just by omitting this or that it really affects how your body works and you can just melt the weight off. And once you get used to it, you don't miss it.'"

Brenda excuses herself to make a quick call home: she's checking up on her kids.

"You must be busy," I observe.

She just laughs and throws up her hands. "My oldest is four and I have a one-year-old. I try to make sure they eat healthy stuff, but they're kids and there are lapses. We do a lot of grilled chicken, I got that from Fight the Fat, and I make them aware of how important it is to put a limit on the candy. I have a huge family—cousins, second cousins, I think I'm related to almost everyone in the area—and a lot of them are in it. I went to school with these people. They are my teachers and my friends from high school. And they're married and I know their husbands and their children.

"And it's just unbelievable how many people have joined. The nurses at the hospital, the people in the restaurants, even the firefighters' wives are part of it! It's massive; not only in this town, but also in the surrounding communities. A lot of Fight the Fat teams will come in after the meeting and they'll say, 'I gotta be sure I eat healthy tonight!' You can see they're really *up* after the meetings. They really enjoy being a part of it. That's why they're repeats—they keep it up year after year.

"I like to hear their stories and I like to see them change. I don't have time to go to the meetings—my husband is a truck driver; he goes over the road and is gone all week. I have a baby-sitter, an in-home day care, and I feel that as it is, I'm away too much. But a lot of Fight the Fat ideas, many of the lessons sink in anyway. People come in here and say we learned this or that tonight. One thing you'll hear over and over is, 'I have three kids (or four or five) and *I'm glad* it's tonight. I *need* to get away from the kids. I wouldn't do it for anything else. But for my health, I know I'm entitled.' And the thing is, after a while, Fight the Fat helps them get out for other things too! They break a cycle."

The irony is that at the time of interview, Brenda had *not* planned on joining herself. But then she realized she was depriving herself of a great source of support and though it was difficult, she finally joined. And what's more, at the end of the 2001 Fight the Fat she won the prize for having lost the most weight—thirty-seven pounds in ten weeks.

"Could you give me an example of a sandwich you'd recommend—and the way you'd prepare it?" I asked.

"Sure. For less than seven grams of fat, you can have a vegetable sandwich, or vegetables with turkey; a turkey-ham sandwich; roast beef; roasted chicken, either hot or cold—you'd be amazed at the variety. If you like cheese, you can still get the one slice of cheese instead of two. If you've got to have that mayo, maybe you shouldn't put on the cheese but stick just to the mayo. I'll ask, 'Do you really want the cheese today, or are you going for the mayo?'"

Even before she joined Fight the Fat, Brenda was an honorary member, a *secret teammate*—people could feel that she was rooting for them. Her attitude was just as important as her advice, but her advice was right on target too. Since she understood the Fight the Fat way, she even helped people "cheat a little"—people had to shift their eating patterns in a way that was easy, that was gradual, and, most important, that would last. And people responded to Brenda because she cared, she noticed, and they were *ready* to be noticed, to be cared about, and to be supported: Fight the Fat had made them open to that.

The point is, you can find your inspiration *everywhere,* if only *you choose* to look for it. It's possible to know all about nutrition and exercise, to be an expert at all the techniques of dieting and still *do nothing about it* as far as you yourself are concerned. That's where motivation comes in. A person like Brenda, or a good inspirational speaker, can make you *feel the truth of* what you know. You experience it in your gut as well as your mind. And when that happens, you act on it.

There were many exceptional speakers during the Fight the Fat campaign who helped motivate members in just this way.

"Here's a hundred dollar bill!" one of them cried during a Dyersville meeting, holding the money in the air. "Who wants it?"

Hands went up.

"Who *really* wants it?"

People waved their hands and pointed to themselves.

This went on until finally someone got up and took it.

The speaker had made her point.

Your Workbook

The Bulletin Board

Get rich slow! In an article on how to get rich, one item listed by Dwight Lee and Richard McKenzie was to stay healthy! Their research indicated that "a twenty-two year old who exercises an hour a day could be worth an additional two hundred and fifty thousand dollars at retirement, thanks to lower medical bills and a longer career." A quarter of a million dollars is nothing to sneeze at, but fewer expenses are just the tip of the iceberg (lettuce). Another benefit is a richer life!

> "Change is the one thing that will always remain in our lives!"
> — Fight the Fat anti-stress slogan

> "Sow an act, and you reap a habit. Sow a habit, and you reap a character. Sow a character, and you reap a destiny."
> —Charles Reade

> "The body never lies."
> —Martha Graham

What ten quotes have you found the most inspiring in your life? List them.

Some Thoughts on Aging

> "Old age is like everything else. To make a success of it, you've got to start young!"
> —Fred Astaire

America has put so much emphasis on being young that age has become something to be feared, shunned, and disguised at any cost. It is empowering both for younger and older people to consider positive images of what is possible at *any* age.

"It used to be said that you're too old to exercise. Well, the truth is that you're too old *not* to exercise. Most of what passes as aging really isn't—it's disuse."
—Walter Bortz, M.D., associate professor of medicine at Stanford University
and author of *Dare to Be* 100. Dr. Bortz, age seventy, lifts weights, runs,
and as of 2000 had completed twenty-nine marathons!

"How old would you be if you didn't know how old you were?"
—Satchel Paige

http://www.npr.org/programs/morning/100years.html is a great site with stories of centenarians. Abraham Goldstein, a 101-year-old professor, finds time to walk one mile every day. Another profile is of Sadie and Gilbert Hill, both one hundred years old and married since 1920. Researchers at Harvard University's New England Centena/rian Study say the chances of a married couple *both* reaching that age are one in six million—you can beat the odds. Sadie and Gilbert say they aren't sure how they accomplished this, but part of the answer might lie in the fact that they still go dancing together.

"Old age is like climbing a mountain. You climb from ledge to ledge.
The higher you get, the more tired and breathless you become,
but your views become more extensive."
—Ingrid Bergman

In 1565, Spaniards landed at what is now St. Augustine, Florida. One of their goals was to discover the fountain of youth. Imagine what they would they think if they saw what many of our middle-aged folks (sixty to eighty) are doing today? They would surely suppose we had discovered that fountain of youth, and of course we have: it is physical exercise!

> "If you live long enough, the venerability factor creeps in; you get accused of things you never did and praised for virtues you never had."
>
> —I.F. Stone

Your Journal

If you have a food diary, that is, if you've been writing down everything you've been eating, this week's exercise should be easier. Take a long, hard look at your food patterns. That is, go over your daily lists and see which foods meant what to you. After which meals did you feel particularly satisfied? Which foods set off the old out of control cravings? Which foods made you feel comforted? Which foods were so unsatisfying that you ended up wanting more?

After certain meals you *felt like going out and doing more*—you were ready for a walk or a run; you were eager to get back to work. After other meals you *felt like* collapsing onto the couch. You felt tired and bloated. Since these reactions are such a particular combination of psychological and physical responses, you and only you can chart them. By using your journal, you can get a good sense of what will happen the next time you reach for a graham cracker with peanut butter or sit down to a turkey dinner.

Healthy Habit for the Week

Forget that after-dinner nap! Turn your body into a roaring furnace and throw your fat in! Timing can maximize weight loss! What do sumo wrestlers do to gain weight? Easy—they take a huge meal just before they go to sleep. How about reversing the sumo pattern? After you eat, instead of *decreasing* your metabolic rate by resting, why not *increase your ability to burn calories with some exercise?*

It's also a good idea to eat *something*—we're not talking a twelve-course banquet here—after you exercise. Why? Because after you exercise your metabolism revs up and you get a big caloric burn. You're using up calories quickly. If you eat an apple or a cup of yogurt then, the thermic effect of food causes the resting metabolic rate to increase even more. It's a winning combo!

Reward for the Week

What about those "sleepy" societies where they nap in the middle of the day...after a long, refreshing lunch! Forget it—try bringing a pillow to work—are you crazy? But, you can still give yourself an hour every day this week that is your time. For one week, skip that frantic rush around during your lunch hour to take care of things—squeeze in your shopping, pay bills, make calls to your plumber, your dentist, your contractor! If you're at home all day, so much the *worse*. You don't even get a lunch hour (people who work from their homes, stay-at-home moms, caregivers, and others in a similar position tend to grab five minutes here and there for themselves, but don't see to it that they get the block of time they need to *calm down!*).

See how you feel at the end of the week. Sit down and *write out* the benefits—just what was interrupted by your hour for yourself and how you managed afterwards. Maybe we can learn something from those siesta-taking, long-lunch societies!

Team Activity for the Week

Act out! There's nothing like playing out a scene from your life to give you perspective! Take a scene from your life that you find troubling—maybe an interaction that led you to overeat; maybe a visit with a "food pusher" you find difficult to refuse; maybe simply a situation where you always come away feeling bad—and act it out with your teammate(s).

It's amazing how much perspective you'll get just from watching yourself or replaying a scene in your life. Psychologists have used theater therapy in group therapy sessions; it has also been used in prisons and in schools. Why not apply it to weight loss? The principles are the same. You need to relive a troubling experience to understand it: by reenacting it, you are going through the same emotions you had the first time, but since it is "only" a play, you have the distance to understand what's going on, to come to terms with it better, to work it out.

An anonymous member tried it out with a teammate and had this to say, "We took two scenes from our lives, one from hers and one from mine. What was interesting was that the scenes had certain similarities. In some ways she and I are very much alike and have some of the same hang-ups. We got together in the privacy of my basement—everyone else in the house was cordially *not invited*—and we improvised. I mean, I explained the basic situation to my teammate but we decided to wing it, to say whatever came into our heads. And what shocked me were the words that came out of my mouth! I had no idea that this was what I must have *really* been thinking."

Play-acting loosened her up and put her in touch with some of the feelings that she had not dealt with up until then. It's a great exercise for loosening inhibitions and trying out how *the new you* will be in a wide range of social situations.

Okay! Curtain! Lights!

Golden Rule for the Week

All weight control experts agree: if you have more than you plan to eat once in a while, on a holiday or special occasion, or even by mistake for no special reason at all, don't think about it. Don't obsess. It's done. Move on. Frequently, those small slips don't matter as much as the guilt or frustration they produce. These psychological after-effects of overeating can do more harm than the overeating itself. The main thing is to keep your morale up and to keep going. Over a long period of time, a few slip-ups every now and then won't matter.

Foods of the Week

Olive Oil. In some towns in Italy they put it on your head after a hair cut! But olive oil is more effective in food where studies show that extra virgin olive oil is effective at keeping LDL (bad cholesterol) from oxidizing. Dr. Ella Haddad says, "We believe that white blood cells pick up only oxidized LDL and deposit it in the artery lining." Regular use of olive oil also dramatically reduces your risk of rheumatoid arthritis.

When you buy it, make sure that the bottle is labeled "extra virgin" (first pressing) or "virgin" (second pressing) since the others have often been extracted from the olives with heat or chemicals. For your health as well as your looks, keep away from deep-fried food in restaurants—they keep reusing the oil, building up levels of oxidized compounds to dangerous levels. Oil that's opened should be kept in the fridge; reheated oil should be thrown out. Oil heated to the point of smoking is highly carcinogenic. Don't overheat when you stir-fry. Even just breathing in the vapors is unhealthy.

Another good oil choice is canola (AKA rapeseed) oil. Buy it "expeller pressed" or "cold pressed" at health food stores and make sure that they're "organic" to avoid the pesticide residues present in ordinary rapeseeds.

Tofu and Soy Protein. These are great sources of low-fat protein that can be used in thousands of creative ways. In Asian restaurants, look out for deep-fried forms of tofu—they're just putting the fat back into a naturally good food. If you see the tofu floating in greasy sauces at the salad bar, forget it. Instead, cut it up and add it to your stir-fry when you're cooking veggies, or add a little soy sauce—your meal will be light and energy-giving.

Here are some great tofu and soy ideas:

A Philippine Treat: Avocado Frappé

Soy milk substitute for condensed milk

¼ ripe avocado

2 tbsp. brown sugar

4 ice cubes

2 tsp fresh lime juice

1) Place ingredients in blender.

2) Blend until smooth.

300 calories per serving

FDA studies find that at least twenty-five grams of soy protein a day can reduce the risk of heart disease. Try hot oatmeal made with cinnamon and soy milk—a great taste!

Try soy sausages and soy bacon! They're tasty and low-fat. And here's another soy treat that may end up becoming a staple:

Soy Scrambled "Eggs"

(Serve hot, like scrambled eggs. Flavor with basil, dill, and chives. Squeezing the tofu will keep the dish from becoming watery.) This recipe is from *Vegetarian Times,* February 2001.

1 lb soft tofu

1 tsp vegetable oil

2 large scallions finely chopped

⅛ tsp ground turmeric

½ tsp salt

6 to 8 medium basil leaves, cut crosswise into fine shreds. (1 tbsp.)

1 tbsp. snipped chives

1 tbsp. finely chopped fresh dill

1 tbsp. finely chopped fresh flat leaf parsley

1) Cut tofu block in half horizontally; then cut in half lengthwise, keeping block intact.

2) One at a time, take a piece of tofu in your hand. Holding it over sink, squeeze tofu gently but firmly until it crumbles slightly and water drips out. When about half the moisture has been removed, place tofu in bowl. Repeat until all tofu has been squeezed.

3) In nonstick skillet, heat oil over medium high heat.

4) Add scallions. Stir just until the sizzle (30 seconds). Add turmeric, salt, and tofu. Stir with wooden spoon, breaking up tofu, until it is evenly golden and moist, about 1 minute.

5) Mix in basil, chives, dill, and parsley. Stir gently until tofu looks like well-set scrambled eggs, about 1 minute. Serve hot.

(122 calories, 5 grams fat)

Self-empowerment Exercise for the Week

Knowledge = power. You want to change your body, your energy level, your mind-set—you've just gotta know what's what! If you don't have the patience to learn nutritional values, or to learn how to read a label (I mean, to really *know* what those percentages mean, to know what the ingredients of the food do for you), *then just think of the payoffs.*

Think of yourself running down the beach in your new bathing suit and feeling super, getting up from a chair without huffing and puffing, or greeting the day with enthusiasm and not with a *God I can't take this anymore* groan—*now* can you take a few minutes to read a label?

And once you get started, you'll find it so fascinating that you'll be telling your spouse over breakfast:

- Did you know that bananas are herbs (the largest around), and that by eating one you are getting only one hundred calories and taking in two of the four fruits you need according to the food pyramid?

- Did you know that fish oil's depression-busting powers make it a great mood food? (Food therapy is very big now! Many new studies are proving the connection between certain foods and certain chemical reactions).
- Did you know that according to a new food discipline called Volumetrics, increasing the amount you eat, the bulk, really helps— so put fruit and vegetables near the top of your shopping list?
- Did you know that after reviewing nineteen other studies, scientists at the University of North Carolina at Chapel Hill concluded that people who put away six cloves of garlic a week are 30 percent less likely to develop colon cancer and about half as likely to get stomach cancer?

You'll be exclaiming to your neighbors, the postman, and your boss at work:

- Did you know that low-fat salsa dips and artichokes are a great snack?
- Did you know that you can have buckwheat or soy noodles instead of white flour for a big boost in nutrition?
- Do you want my recipe for squash soup with corn chowder?
- Did you know that the darkest fruits, those richest in color such as black or red grapes, are richest in antioxidants and help detoxify the body?
- Did you know that lima beans and green peas are terrific sources of protein? (¾ cup lima = 7 grams fat free, body-building protein).

And you'll be giving out tips to cut fat, such as:

- Substitute cocoa for baking chocolate in recipes!
- Try making your hamburger half meat and half pinto beans or black beans for "extra lean mean"—great taste, lots of fiber, and lower fat.

Stress Antidote for the Week

Part of Fight the Fat is trying things you have never tried before, and doing things that *just aren't you,* since part of the way you define yourself is by what you do. I am someone who does this but not that. I watch television, for example, or I take care of my kids—*but I don't do yoga.* Who has time to sit cross-legged looking at your navel? The answer—by now you've probably guessed it with a groan—*you do!* And your teammate(s) will help ease the way because it is much easier to try out something new like yoga or meditation with someone you know and feel comfortable with, and with another beginner like yourself.

"I made all kinds of jokes about it before I tried it," says Carol of Fight the Fat, "but the joke was on me—I love it. Now when I get upset or am having a bad day, instead of fuming or shouting at my kids, I go to my room, close the door, and come out thirty or forty minutes later a new person. My family loves it—especially my son! When I start getting on his case, he says, *Mom, why don't you go do your thing?* And you know what? I do!"

If you live in a large city, you will have the choice of a wide range of yoga teachers, each with different methods. Sometimes people are turned off by one teacher only to be inspired by another. So give it a real try and experiment a while before deciding whether this is for you. You can check out your instructor through the *Yoga Journal*'s Yoga Teachers Directory. Try contacting *Yoga Journal*'s Book and Tape Source, 2054 University Avenue, Berkeley, CA 94704 or logging on to their website: www.yogajournal.com.

Yoga helps you increase the flexibility of your body, teaches you how to breathe, promotes healing through a peaceful mind, and, once you master the basic techniques, can be practiced alone or with a teammate who comes over regularly for a session. While waiting for the laundry to finish or dinner to cook, you can bring more oxygen into your blood stream and stretch your muscles. All for the "price" of trying something new!

In addition to or instead of yoga, there are many forms of meditation. Some have a religious orientation but others are only meant to quiet the mind and body and to make you more receptive to the universe.

The mind never *turns off*—but, the point of meditation is to shift your focus from the endless thoughts that keep distracting you and "quiet" it by focusing on the single object of your meditation—a single word, a single image. It's difficult but if you give it a serious try, you'll see how you feel afterwards. Doubting Thomases invited. Here are a few books on the subject to check out:

- Brenda Shoshanna, Ph.D., *Zen Miracles*
- Lawrence LeShan, *How to Meditate: A Guide to Self-discovery*
- Joan Borysenko, *Minding the Body, Mending the Mind*
- Eknath Easwaran, *Meditation: An Eight-Point Program*

Life is a constant process of widening your horizons, learning new things, and trying new techniques. When life gives you more than you can handle, you have two choices: you can let the pressure overwhelm you, turning that stress into extra pounds and ultimately into diseases like diabetes and high blood pressure. Or, you can release the stress and opt for health.

Let's have a *Hey, I'll do anything it takes* attitude. Because that's what you need if you're going to change your life for good. So get into that half lotus position! Take a deep breath, and start chanting.

Chapter Nine: Handling Others

You can take the house, the car, and the dog—just leave me the Ben & Jerry's!

"Hell is other people!"
—Jean-Paul Sartre

"Sartre could have added, *So is heaven!*"
—Fight the Fat organizer, Dianna Kirkwood

Two Contrasting Husband and Wife Scenarios

I. "After joining Fight the Fat, I knew that I would be away from home more. So, I began showing my husband how much I still cared about him—in small ways, quietly, to offset any pressure he was feeling from my being away. It wasn't just the really nice shirt and cufflinks I got him, or the corn bread I made (he loves my corn bread), but it was all those extra hugs and kisses that told him *No way is this going to be bad for our marriage.*"

II. *She:* "...and another thing! It hurts me when you look at other women when I'm with you—especially when it's my birthday."

He: "You're different since you've been on that diet! I liked the old you more...If you're going to keep on this way—it means trouble..."

You're different—so many Fight the Fat members report having these words hurled at them as an accusation. But *of course* you're different, and thank God for it! Speaking to hundreds of members, I've heard this kind of fight described in one form or another many times. *He's so uncooperative. She's gotten so selfish.* I've also heard of very warm, loving family members who go all out to support the new healthy changes taking place.

The positive situations don't require any work (except to remember to acknowledge and thank those who give you support! Don't take them for granted). So, let's deal with the problems, with the worst-case scenarios. If you're having a *you're different* fight, the issues may not be the same as the ones described above, but it comes down to the same principle: when you succeed in turning around your life, we're talking *change*, and change is threatening. It might be the kids complaining *You're never around at night anymore*—because you take off a night or two for exercise and a meeting. It might be some relative getting on your case during a holiday dinner or a family get-together because you're not cleaning your plate of the high-calorie, fatty food she's cooked *especially for you!* (That's a hard one.)

Or, it might be a husband or boyfriend like Gretta's (not her real name), "Sometimes those nearest to you won't support your change of lifestyle. When I was really heavy and putting on extra pounds every week, my husband kept nagging me to do something about it and even made fun of me. But when I finally did something about it and joined Fight the Fat he said, *You'll never last*—that was my first shock.

"My second shock came when I was really sticking to Fight the Fat. About week seven he screamed at me *All we have to eat in this place is vegetables, there's nothing good in the fridge!* The fridge was packed with lots of great stuff, so I said *If you want junk food, you know where to get it. But don't bring it back, or else it'll get dumped! I don't want it around.* That made him see red! He should have been cheering me on and instead all he could do was gripe. It made me think that all the time he was nagging me about being fat he was just getting off on it. After all, that puts him in a powerful position (that's what one of my team members thought). Here I was the one out of control and he was the healthy one. I don't see any other way to look at it. The new me must be shaking him up."

"How are you dealing with this?" I asked.

"It's good to know, but it's not the end of the world. I was disappointed with his reaction, but I have a whole team behind me, they back me up whenever I need it now."

Another woman in a similar situation said, "You can never tell who will really support you. I don't look to my husband to help me with my weight problem—I look to my team."

This is the *very first* thing to keep in mind. Now you have your Fight the Fat buddy or your Fight the Fat team, whichever it may be, to support you, to compare notes with you, to say to you *You're doing great. Keep going!* You may not think you need to hear this, but you do. Over a long period of time, this kind of support is crucial in counteracting whatever negative feedback you've been getting from others.

Your teammate or teammates, or your Fight the Fat buddy, will confirm *your* reality. She will tell you that there is *plenty* of good food in the fridge, that you have a *right* to live in a temptation-free house, and that it is important to take off whatever time you need for exercise and meetings and stress relief!

The beauty of being part of a Fight the Fat campaign is that you take in the right message about yourself and about what you're doing. We're constantly aware of the way others react to us whether we know it or not. Their attitude and their opinion affect ours. They are our mirrors, and if that mirror is distorted, like the one you see in a fun house, then our self-image gets distorted, too.

Sometimes a single comment can have a tremendous effect on you—for good or bad—especially when it's repeated over and over again. You pick up the attitude. When you've lost ten pounds and have another thirty to go and someone "reminds" you how much you still have to lose, that can throw you off.

And the opposite is also true. Lila of the Dyersville *Finished with Fat* (eight dedicated members) explained how something Bobbi Schell, Mercy's Supervisor of Rehabilitation Outreach Services, "is always saying" finally got through to her. "Bobbi's motto is *Health comes in all shapes and all sizes* and that took the pressure off me. Whenever I tried to lose weight in the past, I was in this great rush. I was under this strain to get it off fast. It didn't make sense, but I felt I had to be thin right away. But after a few weeks, I couldn't take the pressure anymore and quit. Bobbi helped me shift my goal to becoming the best I could be at whatever weight I am. *The pounds will come off if you do the right thing!* she kept saying. And I guess *I finally really heard her.* Now when I can do more on the treadmill or can walk up a flight of stairs without losing my breath, it makes me feel hopeful. And feeling hopeful keeps me going."

Another strength you get from having your reality confirmed is that you become more assertive. You insist on what you need and deserve. The kinds of *you're different now* confrontations described above are bound to take place as you stand up for yourself. After all, you're not blissed out on sugar anymore; you're off your *two, no, three scoops please* tranquilizer.

So, something's got to give! Look at it this way:

Which would you rather do?
1) Confront your husband (wife) or boyfriend (girlfriend) about something that's not right in your relationship.
2) *Eat a piece of cake.*

Which is easier?
1) Telling your boss you're unappreciated at work?
2) Telling your mother or mother-in-law to stop interfering?
3) Telling your sister how upset you were she never thanked you for that sweater you spent months knitting?
4) *Eating a piece of cake?*

Finally, which is less painful?
1) Feeling lonely or sad during the holiday season?
2) Remembering someone no longer in your life?
3) Dealing with serious illness (your own or that of someone close to you)?
4) Feeling really happy about something, and having no one to share it with?
5) *Eating a piece of cake?*

An impossible schedule, a new job, relatives who are too demanding, someone who is taking advantage of you—you've been using food to put up with things that have been too much for you. Now that you're on Fight the Fat, what are you gonna do?

To begin with, you have to figure out your pattern, the way you interact with others and how it affects your eating. At a meeting of an anonymous team ("no names, please"), a team that has been meeting regularly near Dyersville for the last two years to exercise and discuss personal problems, a woman who was a fairly new addition told her teammates, "It's interesting, my husband didn't mind at first. But now he's having a real hard time."

"We've all had to work through this with our husbands," another team member answered her. "I've asked mine to come exercise *with me*. I tell him that I'd love that (and it's true). He doesn't do it, but just my asking stops him from feeling shut out."

"I tell mine," said a third teammate, "think of the kids—it's the best and healthiest thing for me to be doing Fight the Fat. I'll be setting a great example."

"Our husbands were used to having all our time to themselves," the team captain added with a smile. "And now, well, you know, we're looking good. I think they get jealous. We can remind them what they mean to us! That's all mine needs—a little special attention."

These women are talking about their husbands, but you can have problems even with people you know casually. An overweight friend, upset that she is losing an eating partner, or feeling jealous of the new healthy you can get under your skin by saying, "You don't look good, you got too thin!" They can try to shake your self-confidence with a "concerned" remark such as this. And while it may not bother you at the time, sometimes these kinds of barbs have a way of echoing, of coming to mind in a crisis when you need all your will power to stay motivated.

Fight the Fat organizer Bobbi Schell says, "There are always the critics, negative types who enjoy picking on you because they aren't too happy with themselves (who knows what's bothering them, and *who cares!*). It's easier to criticize you than to look in the mirror. They are always there to point out how terrible you look when you are overweight, but they would rather die than give you a compliment when you've shed those pounds and are looking good. But hey, you know how you are doing. And remember, in the long run you are doing it for you!"

Another member says, "My mother-in-law, who was always telling me to lose weight, now started in that I'd gotten too thin! I knew I wasn't too thin, my doctor thought I was at my perfect weight. But I didn't argue with her. I just told her that she was probably right but I couldn't do anything about it since my husband loved me this way! He couldn't get enough of me! That really shut her up!"

One quote that got a big hand of applause when it was read out loud at a Fight the Fat meeting was from Teddy Roosevelt. He had this to say about critics (if he'd lived today he would have said the man *or woman),* "It is not the critic who counts, not the man who points out how the strong man stumbles or where the doer of deeds could have done them better. The credit belongs to the man [or the woman!] who is actually in the arena, whose face is marred by dust and sweat and blood, who strives valiantly, who errs and comes up short again and again because there is no effort without error and shortcomings. Who knows the great devotion, who spends himself in a worthy cause, who at the best knows in the end the high achievement of triumph and who at worst, if he fails while daring greatly, knows his place shall never be with those timid and cold souls who know neither victory nor defeat."

Frances, a Dyersville retiree who is now among the fittest members of the community, has a shorter quote that she uses to silence people she calls *self-esteem snipers,* "If anyone doesn't like me the *new way,* I just repeat something the Duchess of Winsdor said, 'A woman can never be too rich or too thin!'" The Duchess didn't do too badly for herself, as people may remember. She was the *middle-aged woman* the King of England gave up his throne to marry in the 1930s. (While this is a good comeback, it's important to be sensitive to the fact that for some people losing too much weight is just as serious an issue as being overweight. Such people should seek professional help.)

Even people who try to be supportive of your weight loss can be a headache. Not a single Fight the Fat member I interviewed said that she or he joined because of a spouse or a family member's suggestions. Just the opposite; *all* the people I spoke to felt that the "others" should have kept their mouths shut! (Sometimes they put it more politely.) "Advice" or pressure actually made it harder, not easier, to join.

This is because if the decision is going to last, it has to be made by you and you alone. You have to be the one taking control. People who diet to please a nagging spouse or a critical parent, end up doing just that—"dieting." They knock off a few pounds before going back to their old eating patterns. They don't make long-lasting changes in their lives because the inner commitment isn't there. *You're going off your diet with a vengeance today* is a phrase we often hear that may be true.

"If you're dieting to please others, you often end up eating to get back your independence," says Fight the Fat organizer Dianna Kirkwood. "It's great when the others in your life support your decisions. But you must take that first step yourself."

One of the Mercy nurses, a young mother on the *Lifesavers* team (eight caregivers from Mercy Medical Center in Dyersville) had this to say, "My husband is very active, a runner. He's a great guy who really was worried about me so he'd often keep on asking me (especially after we had the children) 'Don't you think it's time we got started here?' But I wouldn't want to hear it—I just wasn't ready yet. You don't want to hear it until you're ready mentally and emotionally. Everybody in the world can tell you that you need it, but it won't matter until something gets to you. I mean, I'm a nurse—I *knew!* I had all the information. I saw what extra weight did to people every time I went to work in the hospital. But I just wasn't ready.

"Fight the Fat got me motivated. I was able to say, *Yes, I will try that. Yes, it's time.* It gave me the extra push. The team effort helped me decide to throw myself into it—after sitting there that first night, listening to Bobbi and the cheering and all, I thought to myself, *Louise, let's go!"*

I asked, "What kinds of changes have you made since joining?"

"Nutritionally speaking, I always knew what to do. You shop around the outside of the supermarket first, of course: fruits and vegetables, then maybe some pasta, Lean Cuisines, that kind of thing. And now that's what I'm actually doing. Another thing is that for me, weighing in weekly was a big deal. At home when I gained a pound, I didn't care as much. Here, knowing a stranger would look at the scale motivated me.

"Another thing I've tried to change is the thought: *I know I'm a good mother and wife if I have this huge spread on the table for the family.* I always used to end up putting up too much food on the table. Before it was meatloaf, mashed potatoes, [and] corn covered with butter. Since I've been on Fight the Fat, it's chicken on the grill, baked potato, tossed salad. I eat at the Ritz, the ostrich is delicious—and lean, really low-fat. Now I order a baked potato with lemon or salsa on it instead of butter or cream. I go for LeRoy's low-fat pizza. It's also very good, the best pizza in town. My mom—who's also in Fight the Fat —cooks separately for herself and for her husband since he's stubborn and impossible!"

It's all about permanence. The kinds of changes Louise made will last a lifetime because she put the pieces of her weight-loss puzzle together *herself,* or with help that *she herself actively sought out when* she *saw she needed it. She* was ready to become motivated. *She* took the steps *she* felt *she* needed. And then *she* made the lasting changes in her life.

Louise tuned out her husband until she was ready. Other members report that this kind of nagging only made them eat more. It was their way of saying to their spouses or children *Love me the way I am.* And of course, the issue isn't love but health! But when someone is very close to you, all kinds of issues become intertwined. That is why you can hear things from strangers that you can't hear from those you live with.

Another category of *significant others,* people who affect us for good or bad, are eating partners! Usually they are overweight friends, and if the two of you are in the habit of eating rich, fattening food together, it's going to be awfully hard to go back to the same restaurant and *watch* them indulge while you have your salad and baked potato. You might do it once, you might do it twice, but after a while it'll become easy to slide back into the old ways.

"A friendship based on food is no friendship," says Cheryl, a Fight the Fat member who transformed herself from a couch potato into a nutrition-conscious woman with a well-toned body. "Of course, I still go out to dinner with friends. But if people want to center their lives around eating, that's up to them—it's not the new me. On a beautiful Sunday afternoon, I'd rather be out hiking now that I'm fit. When the focus of your life changes, the people in your life end up changing, too. It's inevitable. Nobody can drag me back to my old ways, because I tell them these five words, *My health is my priority*, and I mean it."

Some people can "make you" eat even from long distance—at least that's what Pauline tells us. A high school teacher in Dubuque who "woke up one morning with thirty-five pounds to lose," she joined Fight the Fat and shed half of it by the end of this, her first year. "A big breakthrough for me was realizing what got me in trouble. During a Fight the Fat meeting, my teammates and I made a list of every time we had overeaten during that month. For me, it turned out that most of the bingeing took place when I was on the phone with my mother who lives out of state. I'd end up getting into the ice cream, the cake, whatever was around *for the kids.*

"I love my mother, but she's always been tough on me. She's always telling me that I spend too much money, or that I'm not raising my kids right, that kind of thing. So, now I never, never, never talk to her when I'm in the kitchen—that's the first thing. Being in the wrong place at the wrong time definitely makes a difference. I also try to wait until I know I'm up to it. Sometimes I'll have exercised first and I'm feeling in a good mood—you know, strong, ready to take on anything. When it's nice out, I'll take the phone into the garden and lie in the sun while we talk. Or I'll take the phone into the bathtub, although my husband tells me I'm going to get electrocuted one day. For me, it was all about coming up with a plan and sticking to it."

Sometimes the others in our lives don't realize how important certain changes are. They are used to the pattern that has been so disastrous for you and don't understand why it has to change. For example, Gloria, another successful Fight the Fat member who lives just outside of Dubuque, found that she had gotten into the habit of watching television with her husband at night and munching on potato chips, pretzels, and cheese-doodles while taking "sips" from "his" beer.

Her husband could afford it, weight-wise. He was over six feet and does heavy lifting during the day (he drives a UPS truck). And she went along with her husband's eating style without thinking much about it—until she was thirty-five pounds overweight. She still watches television with her husband, but getting a good tip from her teammate, she moved the television into the "back" room where she keeps her stationery bike. Her husband balked at the idea. The "back" room is not as comfortable as the living room; it's hotter in the summer and colder in the winter; and it's further from the kitchen. But she had made up her mind to succeed this time at weight loss and refused to let anything get in the way.

"I said if he wouldn't let me move the television, I'd buy another one for myself. Getting the television wasn't such a big deal, but I liked being with my husband at night. So, I hoped he'd give in. And he finally did when he saw I wouldn't back down." Now she watches television munching on carrots instead of chips and sometimes she bicycles during the commercials, "Not as often as I thought I would, maybe twice a week." But it doesn't matter because when she moved to the back room, she was sending a strong message to herself and to her husband. She was breaking a pattern. She was standing up for her health, her looks, the new her—and that was empowering.

Dianna Kirkwood sums up the importance—and the unimportance—of others well. After helping run her fourth Fight the Fat, she said, "After talking to so many people, I feel like the voice of experience, the combined experience, I mean, of all the members. Let me just make one generalization. *The more important a person is in your life, the more power they have to inspire you or drag you down if you let them.* These last four words—*if you let them*—are so important because that puts the ball back in your court. What you do, what you decide to eat or not to eat, ultimately is up to you."

Your Workbook

The Bulletin Board

"The two most powerful warriors are patience and time."
—Chinese saying

"You want the rainbow, you gotta put up with the rain."
—Dolly Parton

"The lazier a person is, the more they plan to do tomorrow."
—Norwegian proverb

"You've come too far in life to take orders from a cookie!"
—Stephen Gullo, *Thin Tastes Better*

"Great enthusiasm, backed by horse sense and persistence, is the quality that most frequently makes for success."
—Dale Carnegie, *How to Win Friends and Influence People*

"Every saint has a past, and every sinner has a future!"
—Oscar Wilde

Your Journal
Figuring Out Your Patterns

Where? When? Why? I eat after I do what? I eat before I do what? Without thinking about it, you find yourself in the kitchen. Your hands, and your mouth have a will of their own. You are searching through the shelves, eating everything in sight. Why? What's going through your mind? How did you get there?

Use the following questions to track your reactions. Use specific examples from your life. After you are finished, try to see a pattern. Think about it. *Seeing* a predictable pattern is a giant step forward—it's half the battle of self-understanding and self-change.

1) *How do I feel when I stay on track?*

2) *How do I feel when I'm eating out of control?*

3) *How do I feel before exercise?*

4) *How do I feel after exercise?*

5) *When I hear good news, I...*

6) *When I hear bad news, I...*

7) *When I am angry, I...*

8) *When I am in a good mood, I...*

9) *How do I feel when I must buy new clothes because I've lost weight? How do these feelings affect my eating?*

10) *How do I feel when I must buy new clothes because I've gained weight? How do these feelings impact on my eating?*

Healthy Habit for the Week

There's no better way to prevent or minimize injuries to the muscles than by keeping them loose and flexible. When you walk or run, you are pounding on the muscle, "shortening" it, actually. Without a good stretch, the tension remains in the muscle, and over time too much tension leads to injuries. There are special stretches for pregnant women and for the elderly. And there are also special stretches for kids. So, if you want your youngsters to join you (it's a good idea—they'll enjoy it and keep you honest) and they're anywhere from age three to fourteen, make sure you look into their special needs.

The Complete Idiot's Guide to Healthy Stretching by Chris Verna and Steve Hosid is an excellent introduction to this overlooked but crucial activity. Take one example, neck flexibility. "Neck pain is almost always caused by neck flexibility problems with the shoulder sometimes playing a role.

Without moving your shoulders, try to gently touch your ear to your shoulder. Don't force or crack your neck, only go as far as it will comfortably let you." It's a simple movement—but think of how much strain you put on those muscles when you hold the phone to your ear with your shoulder and talk while using your hands to do chores.

Stretching is an activity you can fit in comfortably during the day, while waiting for a bus or elevator, talking on the phone, or standing on line in the supermarket. Learn the proper moves, and by the end of the day your muscles will be saying *Thank God!*

Reward for the Week

In vino veritas.
In wine there is truth!

Wine, that gladdens the heart of man!
—Psalm 104

Studies have shown that one or two glasses of wine may be beneficial to your health—two five-ounce glasses for men, one for women. Wine is believed by many to prevent heart disease (how's *that* for a reason to drink? *I'm doing it on doctor's orders!* That should shut up any critics, and allow you to enjoy a drink guilt-free.). We're talking red wine and more specifically we're talking about wines that contain the *phenol* compounds—that's a catch-all term including the *flavonoids* that have the ability to strengthen your heart. Among the wines tested, the cabernet sauvignon, petite sirah, and pinot noir got the highest grades, according to the *Journal of Agricultural and Food Chemistry*. Need I say more? Toast the new you as you enjoy this week's reward!

Team Activity for the Week

Eating out together—practicing some new skills! Pick a restaurant for a team meal together and plan the outing as carefully as if you were going to a battle (because you are!).

Advice to all Fight the Fat members from Mercy nutritionist Jane Clemen: "If you walk through those restaurant doors starving, chances are you'll walk out of them having overeaten or, let's just say, not having made the best choices. Having had a light snack about a half-hour before, some fruit or a graham cracker with peanut butter, will make you less vulnerable to temptation. If you are eating out, make an effort to study the menu beforehand if possible.

"Don't be shy about asking questions about exactly how the food is prepared. Don't be shy about requesting modifications such as *No mayo, please.* Or, *Can you grill the fish instead of frying it? Can you steam it?* Don't feel that you must eat whatever is put in front of you. Before you begin to eat, measure out what *you* consider is a reasonable portion and put the excess on an extra plate or ask the waiter to put it in a doggie bag.

"Don't *touch* the bread basket before the meal comes—fill up on water instead (most people consume so much bread and butter that they've had an entire meal before the meal). Learn how to eat slowly, and to linger and enjoy the atmosphere as much as the food."

As a group, you can help one another in making the best choices, especially if you're prepared for your outing with a discussion of the do's and don'ts of eating out. Here are some tips.

Best Choice when Eating Out

Mexican
Tostada with veggies.
Plain corn tortillas with Chile sauce.
Avoid tacos and enchiladas.

Japanese

Sushi and sashimi (raw fish).
Steamed fish and vegetable dishes.
Avoid the tempura.

Seafood

All shellfish are high in cholesterol (shrimps, oysters, clams, lobster, etc.), but relatively low in calories if steamed or broiled.
Ask for poached or broiled plain or "dry" baked fish.
Forget the tartar sauce and butter.
Forget anything deep-fried.
Season with lemon and lime and pepper.

Italian

Try the pasta with a vegetable sauce (*primavera* with pasta).
Piccata = Sautéed Plain with Lemon.
Avoid the garlic bread—it's a sure way to start overeating.
Forget the parmigiana; ditto the shrimp scampi.
If they have *zabaglione* you're in luck (200 calories a serving, it's one of God's gifts—it tastes like its 1,000 calories a bite).

Chinese

Soups are okay.
Say *no!* to the fried noodles.
Avoid egg rolls, shrimp, fried rice.
Ask for no MSG, and emphasize that you want only a *little bit of oil* to be used in the preparation of your dish.
The Chinese make spareribs lean, so you can chance it.
Steamed fish Chinese style is delicious.

American *(whatever that means!)*

A small sirloin = 350 calories.

Baked potatoes are good choices if you veto the butter.

Chili has only 300 calories and twelve grams of fat.

Beans are an excellent source of fiber (so think chili & beans).

At the salad bar, skip the high-fat, creamy salad dressings.

Choose greens that are darkest in color for highest nutritional value.

French

Say *Non, merci* to:

Onion soup made with cheese and bread

Anything *rémoulade*—that is made with mayonnaise

Vichyssoise and other cream-based soups

Try fish but make sure you fight shy of the rich sauces.

Fish that's poached or served *a la nage* is a good choice.

A rack of lamb is another lean possibility.

Golden Rule for the Week

In keeping with this week's topic, make it your rule to stop and think. Am I hungry—or am I nervous, bored, tense, unhappy, or mad? Don't use food to deal with non-food situations, such as anger, disappointment, anxiety, or unhappiness.

Weight counselor Dr. Didi Fujita says, "People use food as if it were a drug. If Karl Marx lived in the USA in 2001 he would have said, 'Food is the opiate of the masses! Overweight of the world unite! You have nothing to lose but your chins!'"

Food of the Week

Figs. I give a fig! Classic French presentation: fresh figs on a bed of crushed ice in a fine dish.

A study by the U.S. Department of Agriculture announced that figs provide a feeling of fullness and prevent overeating. Figs are a rich source of calcium, are high in fiber, and are a good natural laxative. Plus they're easy to carry around for a "food emergency."

When you need that extra boost of energy during a slump in your workday, and when you're exhausted from running after the kids or stuck in traffic and late for an appointment, instead of reaching for a chocolate bar, take out two or three figs and eat them *slowly*. Instead of the nutritionally empty snacks you have been consuming, you're promoting good health and preventing a binge later since all that fiber helps you come to the dinner table feeling satisfied, not deprived (two figs give you more fiber than a half cup of beans!).

Get in the habit of including the following in your meals and you have a low-fat and protein-rich alternative to meat. Include these foods in soups, complement them with large salads and desserts of fresh fruit, and you are on the way to success.

Brown rice is preferable to white rice, since it is fiber rich and has not lost its nutritious outer covering. One cup of brown rice gives you six grams of protein.

Beans. More protein than steak! Low-fat! Cheap! Healthy! What more can you ask? Lentils, peas, and dried beans are low in fat and high in protein. Combine beans with a grain (rice, corn, millet, barley, wheat) and you get a *complete protein*—that is, a food with all the amino acids your body needs. A few drops of "Beano," an anti-gas solution sold at health food stores, can solve the problem of flatulence; alternately, the digestive system will adjust quite quickly if you eat beans every day for about a week.

If eaten together, grains plus beans yield 40 percent more protein than if eaten separately. One and a half cups of beans with four cups of rice (keep this proportion) has as much protein as a nineteen-ounce steak.

Self-empowerment Exercise for the Week

Earlier in this book, a notice or two has been included titled *For Those Who Need to Be Scared*. Actually, there is a behavior modification technique called aversion therapy that emphasizes the *negative* consequences of behavior you want to change.

You know that by eating too much, and by not moving except to go to the refrigerator, you are asking for it—"it" being clogged arteries, a heart attack, diabetes, high blood pressure—to name a few diseases you're courting. But the words "at high risk" somehow mean nothing for most people! When they feel the chest pains, when they go into an insulin sweat, then it's real. Now it's just words on a page competing with a very real dessert making our mouths water. It's easy to see which option will win out—especially since we have a way of denying or forgetting what we don't want to think about.

However, by saying "insulin sweat" and "chest pains" just now, I probably got your attention more than if I had stuck to the words "diabetes" and "heart disease." That's because what I began to do was make these conditions more real, more concrete, by describing them. You can continue this process by actively *learning* more about the negative consequences. Visualize what you read about. It will be one hour of your time. Go to the library and take out a few popular medical books written for the general public. Get to understand the process by which overweight, sedentary people are killing themselves. The next time you see a hot fudge sundae, you might "see" a patient sitting next to it!

Stress Antidote for the Week

"The amount of sleep required by the average person
is about five minutes more!"
—Wilson Misner

There is sleep—and then *there is sleep!* Falling asleep with the television blaring the details of the latest murder, taking your work to bed with you, obsessing about tomorrow's meeting or yesterday's late project, sleeping in a room where the alarm clock ticks and the computer screen hums and the phone rings, or in a room that's too warm (sixty to seventy degrees is the optimal temperature) with the pillows under the bed instead of supporting your neck—these are all ways you can miss out on the benefits of a deep, anxiety-free night of peace and renewal.

What are some of the symptoms of sleep deprivation? At the top on the list is reduced motivation. Which means, when you're feeling tired or haven't gotten enough rest, you're at risk for falling into that dangerous *What does it all matter? mood.* Depression, anger, and not feeling up to the day's challenges are other equally destructive states of mind that come to the fore in an exhausted state.

Sugar and chocolate cravings have nothing to do with appetite during these times. You're turning to food to keep you going when what you need is a good night's sleep! Chocolate is a stimulant because it contains not only caffeine but also another chemical stimulant, *theobromine.* Studies done over the last two decades determined that chocolate contained a number of compounds chemically similar to amphetamines. Do you hear that, all you chocoholics out there? Or are you too stimulated, too hyped up to be able to read?

We're not talking calories now! We're talking drugs! The darker the chocolate, the more caffeine there is in it. A one and a half–ounce serving of dark chocolate will have thirty-two milligrams of caffeine; the same serving size of milk chocolate will contain only nine milligrams of caffeine. White chocolate is not even officially chocolate—it contains too little of the material extracted from the cocoa bean. If you're looking to wean yourself off the habit, maybe that's one way to start.

So, if you drink hot cocoa to relax before going to sleep, remember, a typical cup of hot chocolate contains a whopping fifteen milligrams of caffeine plus the other stimulants, which means you're giving your body a loud *Stay awake!* message. The actual stimulant effect of a chocolate product is about *double* the amount of caffeine there is in it.

Dr. Pepper, Mountain Dew, or Sunkist Orange also contain significant amounts of stimulants, usually caffeine. Coca-Cola—the Colas are in a class by themselves!—was concocted in the 1880s by John S Pemberton, a Confederate officer and a pharmacist. Pemberton was looking for a stimulant, and he found it in the cocoa plant from which low doses of cocaine can be extracted and which proved to be ten times more of an upper then caffeine. To this ingredient he added an extract of the African Hell seed, also known as the kola nut, which contained highly concentrated caffeine.

To counteract the kola nut's bitterness, Pemberton then added large amounts of sugar and flavoring—citrus, cinnamon, and vanilla, blended according to a formula so secret that the two people who are in on it are forbidden by the Coca Cola company from traveling together on the same plane. In the event of an accident, this unhealthy, syrupy, addictive drink would be lost to humanity forever! Every twelve-ounce serving of Coca Cola contains around thirty-five milligrams of caffeine. Pepsi contains even more. And Tab wins the contest for worst at forty-four milligrams of caffeine.

People get addicted to Coke or Tab, and they use it for the boost that sleep should give them. Sooner or later, they pay the price in terms of their health and in terms of calories. When they start to "crash" from their caffeine high, they feel depleted and tend to get the munchies (the same reaction goes on when speed or No Doze wears off. You become ravenous).

In any case, an herbal tea is a better preparation for sleep than a Coke, diet or no diet, time for thought and reflection is better than falling asleep to the description of the latest grisly crimes. Turn off that radio or television, open the window a crack, shut the lights, the computers, the phone, and get some sleep so that you can function without your caffeine and chocolate. You owe it to your body.

Chapter Ten: Beginning

"I shall pass through this world but once. Any good therefore that I can do or any kindness that I can show to any human being, let me do it now. Let me not defer or neglect it, for I shall not pass this way again."
—Mahatma Gandhi

"The only way to have a friend is to be one!"
—Ralph Waldo Emerson

"To complete a thing, a hundred years is not sufficient.
To destroy it, one day is more than enough."
—Chinese proverb

"You end up as you deserve. In old age you must put up with the face, the friends, the health, and the children you have earned."
—Fay Weldon

"Let's take care of today and forever will take care of itself!"
—Rosalie Kaufman, author of *Yes You Can!*

"There is no finish line!"
—Nike

Week ten is a kind of contradiction. Despite that Nike slogan, there *is* a finish line and week ten is it! Congratulations, you've arrived! Take time to savor that.

It's important to recognize what you have achieved and celebrate it. Give yourself credit—you deserve it. Take a good long look at where you've come from and think about all the changes you've made from week one until now. *It's taken two and a half months of hard work to create the new you.*

But this is all on the one hand. *On the other hand,* you're not finished yet because creating the new you is a process that really has no end.

To say that you're at the *beginning* does not take away from what you've done. Beginnings are hard. But now it's important to make sure that what has worked for you over the past ten weeks becomes a regular part of your life.

Take the following example from a Chamber of Commerce St. Pat's dinner in Dyersville. As the salad was passed around—together with three rich and rather fattening dressings—*Fight the Fat* organizer Dianna Kirkwood heard a woman remark to her husband, "Do you remember that salad dressing I made when I started Fight the Fat? It had yogurt and ground almonds in it and sesame seeds and was really delicious. I wonder why I never made it again?"

Why didn't she make it again? Simple: call it laziness, the force of gravity, inertia, old habits! If she'd pasted the recipe up on her fridge and used it a few times during the ten weeks of the campaign, her salads would have had more pizzazz—another incentive to eat those greens! *Plus* she would have *reinforced* a good habit she'd formed, namely, eating lots of veggies on a daily basis. It takes focus; and it takes concentration to keep juggling that many balls in the air.

That's where your new Fight the Fat partners come in. Week ten is about you and your teammates renewing your commitment to working with each other. It's about making sure that those great recipes aren't forgotten, that the exhilarating volleyball game doesn't become a once in a lifetime event!

Think of a tennis match or Ping Pong or volleyball game that you've enjoyed during the campaign. It burned off pounds! It got your heart going; it was lots of fun. *Regularly* schedule it into your week. Introduce another angle to the friendly rivalry. If you're a two-member team, try challenging the kids or your spouses once you and your teammate have really gotten good. Punish them! Teach them a lesson, while at the same time getting into *activity*, motion, and movement.

If you're part of a team competition, try making your meets more frequent by setting up a tournament—best three out of five, say, or a *series* of tournaments with a year-end prize. Grownups are like kids that way. They love to play, to compete, to win, and to *almost* win. The "if only I hadn't tripped" stories are also fun to tell. It's the kind of activity that makes you forget about losing weight while you lose it!

You can also carry over this way of thinking to food competitions. A terrific way of both having fun and coming up with ideas is to have a contest modeled on the kind of creative recipes frequently found in the health magazines. The goal is to produce a dinner that can wake you up with its exotic flavor, contrasting textures, and surprising combinations—using low-fat and low-calorie food.

If you're on a two-member team, you and your buddy can still enjoy the excitement of friendly food rivalry—how about bimonthly contests with friends or family members as the judges (keeping who made what a secret, for impartiality's sake)?

The point is to innovate, to set new goals, and to build on what you have accomplished in order to accomplish even more. There's no better way to stay on your toes.

That was the word from veteran members, who were concentrating on the process of fine-tuning. Arriving at the Recreation Center in Dyersville early one morning, I met two women who were helping set up for the big meeting that night. They were ex-couch potatoes who had done so well over the Fight the Fat campaigns that now they were instructors in exercise classes (in addition to holding down full-time jobs).

The first, Linda, has some more weight to lose—something in the neighborhood of twenty pounds, but she has already achieved a great deal in the way of fitness. She has good body tone and is very stretched out and agile.

The other, Susan, a widow with three children, had reached her weight goal though she is in the process of increasing her stamina and muscle tone (Susan, like most other Fight the Fat members, did not reach her goal weight after her first ten weeks. It took her *two* Fight the Fat campaigns including the months inbetween to get down to the weight she wanted to be).

"How did you decide on when to stop losing?" I asked Susan. "Was it how you looked—or some weight the doctor recommended?"

"Actually, I was influenced by something I read in a book," she answered. "For a long time, I was always either going up or down as far as numbers on the scale went. And each time I tried to diet, my goal was to reach the weight I had been for years—before my kids were born. But this time I decided on ten pounds more because of the book I mentioned. The author was saying that we should pick a goal that is realistic, one that we could live with and maintain without torture!

"Her main point was that you can reach any number you want on the scale, but that the real challenge was to maintain it. And that made sense to me, so I decided to try it with an extra ten pounds this time and focus on getting fit instead of losing every last ounce—although the author on the cover of that book looks pretty skinny, let me tell you."

The book Susan read, it turned out, was one recommended by Fight the Fat organizers, Rosalie Kaufman's *Yes You Can!*, which goes on to say this about long-term weight control, "There's a story about three old men, seventy, eighty, and ninety years old, sitting on a park bench when a pretty young girl walks by. The seventy-year-old says, 'If I were young again, I'd hug her all night.' The eighty-year-old says, 'If I were young again, I'd kiss her all night.' The ninety-year-old says, 'If I were young again—what was that nice thing we used to do?' When motivation goes, we can't even remember all the *nice things* we used to do for ourselves.

"When people fail to maintain their weight loss it is because they stop being important to themselves—they stop putting their own well-being first and let themselves become overwhelmed by worry and grief."

This advice applies across the boards for week ten members, whether you're at your goal weight or still have a way to go. By the time you're two and a half months into the program you need to *remember and repeat* all those "nice things" you did for yourself at the start of the program.

Long-term success means shifting the focus from what you can't eat, and what you shouldn't do, to what you now love to eat, and what you love to do!

A grim, clenched fist, locked jaw attitude—a do or die struggle—can't be maintained for a lifetime. A *Hey, this is fun! This is really delicious and healthy!* philosophy can.

Talking to Fight the Fat members, I heard endless ways that they achieved this kind of long-term success. One of them, Juliette, captain of Dubuque's ten-member team, *The New You,* was particularly smart in thinking up a long-term strategy. Putting her head together with two teammates, the three of them ganged up on their husbands.

"I bought my husband a mountain bike and nagged him to death until he agreed to go out with us on Sundays," she told me. "He didn't need to lose weight, but boy was he out of shape! He'd never listened to me before, but when I told him that we were *all* counting on him—that my teammates' husbands were doing it too!—he finally gave in. I think he didn't want to be the only one left out."

"Do you still all go out together?" I asked.

"Sometimes we do, and sometimes it's just me and my husband. Either way, though, it's become part of our weekends since we *both* really enjoy it (*now* he thanks me for pushing him). Last week we put our bikes on the car and drove an hour or so to a really beautiful place near the river. It's a lot of fun planning where we'll go to bike and I love the fact that we share these long rides together. We have two teenage boys—but they're too lazy!"

Juliette and her teammates knew that by getting their husbands into the picture, they would be increasing their chances of long-term success. They just didn't give up until they'd succeeded. And the fact that they acted together helped convince their spouses.

Whatever the method, the most successful members all had this in common: they took a good, long look at their life patterns and they figured out a way to make exercise a permanent part of it. Jean, a secretary in Dubuque, bought a golden labrador retriever and made the kids promise *not* to walk it. Laura, a cook at Divine Word College in Epworth, switched from playing cards during her breaks to power walking with a coworker she'd convinced to join Fight the Fat.

"The brothers are always encouraging me to use what I've learned at Fight the Fat when I make meals here," she added, "which makes me really happy since so many people can benefit from what I've learned."

Another big benefit of getting into exercise is that you can use this new strength of yours around holiday times. Since the holidays often throw many people, demoralizing them for days or weeks (*before* and after), a really important part of thinking *long-term* is to plan for them.

A threesome that kept going long after the ten weeks were over, calling themselves *We're Doin' It,* called each other in the middle of the afternoon on Thanksgiving—a quick, two-minute call to give each other a shot of support in the midst of all that temptation. That was the first year. The second year they got even more revved up for Christmas, a holiday they all found hard.

Since the team was composed of three young mothers who were also neighbors, they used what they *already* had in place—they jogged together twice a week—to meet the holiday challenge. They decided to meet early on Christmas morning for an extra long jog before the big dinner.

Chris, the member of the team who had the most trouble with the holidays, started brainstorming with her teammates a month before Christmas. "We went back and forth. There's no way we're going to meet Christmas morning. Everyone's going to be busy, everyone's going to be thinking about other things—usually the kids jump into the bed and wake me up and drag me over to the tree. But there's no other time to do it that day. Finally Joan, she lives just down the block and started with me on the *Nevermore Fat* team, said, 'It's only forty-five minutes! Let's just do it! It'll start the day right.'

"And the minute she said that, I knew she was right. Christmas is always a problem because you sit around and talk and eat so much that the next day you're out of it. I mean, what's the point of being careful about what you eat if the day before you blew it with eggnog and all kinds of stuff like that? Christmas always used to be *the end* for me. So, I figured, I'll try anything that'll help. And it was a great idea. We jogged together and gave each other a big hug afterwards—I know this will sound crazy, but that run felt like part of the holiday spirit somehow. I started the day feeling so good about myself that I didn't go crazy eating for once!"

The run was a good idea for many reasons, emotional as well as physical ones. And the holidays are not just a problem because all those rich foods are associated with them—they are an emotional roller coaster as well. The other side of all that holiday joy is a special sadness we experience at this time.

We all feel the passing of time. We remember other holidays when we were kids. We miss our childhood. We think of relatives who are not present. We meet with family members, sometimes siblings we have not seen for a long time, and together fond memories, old jealousies, and grievances are revived. There is a pressure to be happy on holidays. If we are going through a difficult time in our lives, we therefore feel our problems doubly. Which is why the suicide rate goes up during the holiday season—and why people turn to food.

Stephen P. Gullo, author of *Thin Tastes Better,* says, "What are our terms of endearment? Honey, cookie, sweetie...even in Ghana, the verb *to eat* is used by certain tribes when referring to sex, the expressions of food and love blending until they are indistinguishable."

In going for that early morning Christmas run, Chris was bonding with her teammates *emotionally*—she was facing the day *together* with them. And she was also working off the stress that she felt about resisting temptation. A forty-five-minute run *not only* burned up the extra calories she might take in, but it also prepared her mentally for the day. Not to mention the fact that getting up early in freezing weather on a day off and jogging for forty-five minutes boosted her self-esteem. It gave her an *I can do anything I try* attitude and strengthened her commitment to her Fight the Fat achievement.

Pam, the third member of the Dubuque *The New You* trio, said, "What I liked about it…is the feeling that the three of us were pulling together. It reminded me of the time when I was a girl and my father had a back operation and he couldn't put the crops in. His brother got the neighbors together; they came with their equipment and got the fields all prepared in one day. Working with my team felt the same way. We were all trying our best not only for ourselves but to help each other. Knowing I was helping Chris…made the day very special for me and strengthened me too."

Along with having the technique of exercise, the team members also had their journals in which they could work through their holiday anxieties and fears. Chris, for one, had been journaling every day since the beginning of Fight the Fat to get in touch with her feelings. This kind of focus and attention gave her the ability to experience her holiday sadness rather than just to feel hungry or food deprived. And she also had an arsenal of low-fat recipes and low-fat versions of holiday "fatteners" so that she didn't have to sit by while everyone else was eating.

It doesn't matter whether it's Christmas or the Fourth of July, Thanksgiving or Hanukah, there is always *some* way to prepare a menu that is in keeping with the holiday spirit while staying within Fight the Fat guidelines. Take the following holiday recipe passed around by Fight the Fat members during Thanksgiving last year from *Prevention Magazine.*

Cranberry Pear Relish

3 cups cranberries
2 firm pears, peeled and cubed
1 orange, peeled and cut into ¼-inch slices
½ cup diced sweet onions
½ cup apple cider vinegar
¼ cup honey
2 tbsp. lime juice
1 tbsp. grated lime rind (optional)
1 tbsp. mustard seeds

1) In a heavy three-quart enameled or stainless steel saucepan, combine all ingredients.
2) Bring to a boil over medium high heat. Reduce the heat to medium and simmer, stirring frequently, for thirty minutes or until thickened.
3) Cool to room temperature, then refrigerate. May be prepared up to two days ahead.

(95 calories, 0.6 grams fat)

Turkey is one of the leanest meats, and with this relish you have an irresistible, healthy main course for Thanksgiving. Sweet potatoes are a great source of beta-carotene and satisfying for your sweet tooth. If you cut the butter, marshmallows, and stuffing (which is the point of this recipe, to replace the high-calorie dishes with really tasty, really low-calorie ones) you can come away from the Thanksgiving table satisfied—and slim.

What is true of the holidays is also true of any special event such as a wedding or a birthday celebration. Fight the Fat gives you resources and tools that enable you *to cope* with life—period. If you work at it conscientiously on a day-to-day basis, the holidays and the big family bash can be, well, a piece of cake.

Taking Stock

Ten weeks have gone by! You have acquired new tools, from bok choy to yoga; you've danced and gardened and pumped iron with the best of them. If you look at the checklist at the end of the chapter, you will find a quick summary of the Fight the Fat challenge. By now these are more than mere words on a page to you. They are the wise rules you have begun to live by.

Mercy Supervisor of Rehabilitation Outreach Services, Bobbi Schell, put it this way at the close of last year's Fight the Fat, "As far as I'm concerned, what the word *fat* really stands for in Fight the Fat is a self-destructive lifestyle, a vicious cycle that must be broken. Our program points people in the right direction. It makes them think of their health as well as their looks, the quality of their life as well as their waist size! It gives them vigor and energy and, most important of all, it gives them hope!"

Sarah, the mother of two young children, lost thirty-six pounds and became an excellent swimmer in the bargain. "Last week I was watching my neighbor play with her kids on a beautiful spring day," she told me. "They were tossing a Frisbee back and forth and she was keeping up with them—running even faster than they were. And suddenly I realized with a shock—it was like something had clicked in my head—*I can do that now!* I didn't have to sit on the porch watching and feeling miserable and eating pints of ice cream. I could be a complete person again."

Life is too wonderful not to be lived to the fullest.

Week Ten Checklist

Remember when you get discouraged, you are not alone in this struggle to turn yourself around. Don't be too proud to call a teammate or exercise buddy. You will be helping yourself, and your buddy, at the same time. This is *the key*. This is what makes this time different from the others.

Success is personal. It is different for different people.

Life is about choices. You may make good choices or bad choices, but the bad choices don't make you bad.

Use a journal (written or recorded) every day to keep track of your eating, exercising, and the way you feel.

Set realistic goals of a one-or-two pound weight loss per week.

Be specific about how you will reach your weekly goal—dropping a snack, reducing portion sizes, increased exercise, etc.

Look for problem areas in your daily habits and game plan from there.

Use your journal to vent. This may help you discover what triggers overeating.

Develop skills for a lifetime of success.

Don't put food favorites totally off limits; just reduce frequency and portion size.

No self-starvation. Eating regularly throughout the day will prevent feelings of hunger and help you control amounts eaten.

Modification of eating habits means adapting a lower-fat, lower-calorie eating pattern including normal foods that can be eaten for a lifetime.

No diets. Those who succeeded in losing weight for good did not see themselves as being on a diet, which is by definition a temporary change in eating habits and feels like deprivation. Instead, they made gradual, moderate diet and exercise changes that they viewed as permanent, part of a "new them." Fad diets do not work because they do not get at the heart of the matter: changing unhealthy eating habits.

Moderate exercise, three or more times a week is a key! The important point is to find something you enjoy and can work into your lifestyle.

Eight glasses of water daily. Sometimes we mistake dehydration for hunger.

Do it for yourself. Most people failed to lose weight when they did it for some outside reason—for example, to look good at their wedding or high school reunion. They succeeded when they lost weight for themselves and no one else.

Once again, look at your overall eating pattern. Have you adapted an eating pattern that puts you at risk nutritionally? Are you including foods from all food groups? What groups are you missing? How can you include them in your eating habits?

Live and learn. Every person successful at weight loss has failed on several previous diets. Instead of seeing themselves as failures, they analyzed their reasons for regaining weight and drew valuable lessons from those experiences.

Make time for yourself.

Plan and prepare your food in advance. Know where you will be around mealtimes and make sure you're not stuck in a no-win situation.

Don't weigh yourself more frequently than once a week, and don't let the scale dictate your self esteem! Even though you still have weight to lose, celebrate each success as it comes (like dropping two clothing sizes).

Don't grocery shop when you are hungry. Take the edge off your hunger first with a snack. Then you'll be more likely to make good choices.

Allow people to help you without feeling guilty, unworthy, or dependent.

Lighten up in your mood and you'll shed those pounds! As the saying goes, *Angels take themselves lightly—that's why they fly.*

Small changes make big differences. Focus on one or two issues a week for small cumulative changes that will add up to a new way of eating and thinking. Consider eating that baked potato with no-fat sour cream or low-fat cottage cheese. Consider that short walk after dinner. Take the stairs instead of the elevator. These things add up!

Get rid of those elastic waistlines.

Set new short-term goals for getting healthy as you reach your initial ones.

Remember, *If you think you can't, you won't. If you think you can, you will.*

Think portion size. Even too much healthy food can cause weight gain.

Don't look at one meal or one day. Balance over time brings success.

Look for opportunities to use more energy. Do your own house cleaning. Take a fifteen- to thirty-minute walk after lunch and dinner today. Take a two-minute walk during every commercial break. Physical activity will help you cope with stress and improve your self-esteem. Muscle burns fat and exercise builds muscle. Let's walk.

Reward every effort and every accomplishment.

Don't quit! You will miss the results if you do. So, just don't quit!

Some bad habits can't be changed, but I can learn to manage them.

Remember: my self-esteem does not depend on the event of the moment. The scenery changes but my worth remains the same.

More people die in the United States from too much food than from too little.

Resolve: I will pay attention to how my daily habits affect my health.

Find every occasion to have a good laugh today.

Remember: motivation is what got you started. Good habits are what will keep you going.

Recipes

Here are some examples of how Fight the Fat modifies some popular, everyday recipes. As you can see, the changes don't have to be big ones to pay big dividends. Over time, these simple switches will save you thousands of calories.

Ravioli Casserole

Original Recipe
16 ounces spaghetti sauce
One 16-ounce bag frozen mini ravioli
One pound ground beef
8 ounces shredded mozzarella cheese
10 ounces frozen chopped spinach, thawed and squeezed dry
½ tsp salt
¼ cup Parmesan cheese, divided
(556 calories, 32 grams fat)

Healthy Recipe
Use reduced-sodium sauce
One 16-ounce bag frozen mini ravioli
½ pound lean ground beef
8 ounces shredded mozzarella
10 ounces frozen chopped spinach, thawed and squeezed dry
¼ cup Parmesan cheese, divided
(437 calories, 19 grams fat)

1) Preheat oven to 350° F.
2) In an 8-inch square baking pan, place 1 cup of spaghetti sauce; top with half the frozen ravioli, half the ground beef, half the mozzarella cheese, half the spinach, and 2 tablespoons Parmesan cheese.
3) Repeat layering.

4) Bake uncovered, until the ravioli are hot and cheese is golden, 35–40 minutes.

5) Let stand 15 minutes before serving.

Makes 6 servings.

Pumpkin Cake Bars

Original Recipe

4 eggs

1 pound canned pumpkin

1 cup sugar

½ tsp salt

1 tsp ginger

1 tsp cinnamon

¼ tsp cloves

18.5-ounce yellow cake mix

⅓ cup melted butter

(178 calories, 7 grams fat)

Healthy Recipe

2 eggs + 2 egg whites

1 pound canned pumpkin

¾ cup sugar

Omit salt

1 tsp ginger

1 tsp cinnamon

¼ tsp cloves

18.5-ounce yellow cake mix

⅓ cup melted margarine

(165 calories, 6 grams fat)

1) In medium bowl beat eggs, egg whites, pumpkin, sugar, salt, ginger, cinnamon, and cloves together.

2) Coat 13"x 9" pan with vegetable cooking spray.

3) Pour in pumpkin mixture.

4) Combine melted margarine and dry cake mix. Sprinkle over top of pumpkin mixture.

5) Cover with aluminum foil and bake at 325° F for 40 minutes.

6) Remove foil and bake for an additional 40 minutes.

7) Cut into squares and serve.

Makes 24 bars.

Turkey Burger

Original Recipe

1 pound ground turkey

½ cup seasoned breadcrumbs

⅓ cup chopped onion

1 egg

1 tsp soy sauce

1 tsp Worcestershire

½ tsp garlic salt

¼ tsp dry mustard

(365 calories, 18 grams fat)

Healthy Recipe

1 pound ground turkey breast

4 slices whole wheat bread, shredded

⅓ cup chopped onion

2 egg whites

1 teaspoon Worcestershire

½ teaspoon garlic powder

¼ teaspoon dry mustard

(197 calories, 3 grams fat)

1) In a large bowl, combine all ingredients and mix well.

2) Shape into four patties.

3) On a lightly greased broiling pan, broil burgers about six inches from heat three to four minutes per side or until no longer pink inside. (Alternately, burgers may be grilled.) Serve on buns.

Makes 4 servings.

Baked Lasagna

Original Recipe

1 lb pork sausage

1 clove garlic, minced

1 tbsp. parsley flakes

1 tbsp. basil

1½ tsp salt

1 1-pound can (2 cups) tomatoes

2 6-ounce cans tomato paste

10 ounce lasagna or wide noodles

3 cups creamed cottage cheese

2 beaten eggs

2 tsp salt

½ tsp pepper

2 tbsp. parsley flakes

½ cup grated Parmesan cheese

1 lb Mozzarella cheese

(391 calories, 24.6 grams fat)

Healthy Recipe

1 lb extra lean group beef (9 percent fat)

1 clove garlic, minced

1 tbsp. parsley flakes

1 tbsp. basil

Omit salt

1 1-pound can (2 cups) tomatoes
2 6-ounce cans tomato paste
10 ounce lasagna or wide noodles
3 cups 1 percent-fat cottage cheese
2 egg whites
Omit salt
½ tsp pepper
2 tbsp. parsley flakes
½ cup grated Parmesan cheese
1 lb low moisture part skim milk mozzarella cheese
(291 calories, 12 grams fat)

1) Brown meat slowly, drain well.
2) Add next 6 ingredients.
3) Simmer uncovered 30 minutes stirring occasionally.
4) Cook noodles in boiling water until tender, drain. Rinse in cold water.
5) Meanwhile, combine cottage cheese with egg whites, seasonings, and Parmesan.
6) Place half the noodles in 13" x 9" x 2" baking dish, spread half the cottage cheese mixture over. Add half the Mozzarella cheese and half the meat sauce.
7) Repeat layers.
8) Bake at 375° F for 30 minutes. Let stand 10-15 minutes before cutting in squares. Makes 12 servings.

Tuna Noodle Casserole

Original Recipe
1 8-ounce package noodles
1 7-ounce can tuna
1 can cream of mushroom soup
1 tbsp. margarine

1 cup corn flakes, crushed
1 4-ounce can mushrooms
(457 calories, 15.3 grams fat)

Healthy Recipe
1 8-ounce package noodles
1 7-ounce can tuna packed in water, drained
1 can Healthy Request cream of mushroom soup
Omit margarine
1 cup corn flakes, crushed
1 4-ounce can mushrooms
(351 calories, 4.3 grams fat)

1) Cook noodles in boiling water for 20 minutes, then drain off water.
2) Add other ingredients.
3) Pour into 2-quart casserole dish sprayed with vegetable oil spray.
4) Bake in oven at 350–375°F for 45 minutes.
Makes 4 servings.

Cheesy Hash Browns

Original Recipe
2 lb frozen hash browns
½ cup melted margarine
½ cup chopped onion
1 tsp salt
1 can cream of chicken soup
¼ tsp pepper
1 cup sour cream
1 cup 2% milk
2 cups shredded cheddar cheese
2 cups corn flake crumbs

¼ cup melted margarine
(371 calories, 28.5 grams fat)

Healthy Recipe
2 lb frozen hash browns
Omit margarine
½ cup chopped onion
Omit salt
1 can Healthy Request cream of chicken soup
¼ tsp pepper
1 cup nonfat sour cream
1 cup skim milk
1 cup shredded reduced fat cheddar cheese
2 cups corn flake crumbs
Omit margarine
(214 calories, 9 grams fat)

1) Spray 9" x 13" inch dish with vegetable pan spray.
2) Mix thawed hash browns, onion, pepper, cream of chicken soup, sour cream, milk, and cheese.
3) Sprinkle with corn flake crumbs.
4) Bake at 350° F for 1 hour, covered. Can uncover last 10 minutes or until browned. Makes 12 servings.

Chicken & Rice Dinner
Original Recipe
1 tbsp. vegetable oil
4 boneless, skinless chicken breast halves
1 can cream of chicken soup
1½ cups water
¼ tsp paprika
¼ tsp pepper

1½ cup uncooked Minute Rice
2 cups fresh or frozen broccoli flowerets
(437 calories, 12 grams fat)

Healthy Recipe
Vegetable pan spray
4 boneless, skinless chicken breast halves
1 can Healthy Request cream of chicken soup
1 ½ cups water
¼ tsp paprika
¼ tsp pepper
1 ½ cups uncooked Minute Rice
2 cups fresh or frozen broccoli flowerets
(380 calories, 5.3 grams fat)

1) Instead of using oil, spray skillet with pan spray.
2) Add chicken and cook until browned.
3) Remove chicken.
4) Add soup, water, paprika, and pepper.
5) Heat to a boil.
6) Stir in rice and broccoli.
7) Top with chicken.
8) Season chicken with additional paprika and pepper.
9) Cover and cook over low heat 5 minutes or until done.
Makes 4 servings.

Other Suggestions
A sandwich can cost as little, calorie wise, as a light snack!

Grilled Sandwich
Butter-flavored spray
2 slices whole wheat bread

reduced fat cheddar cheese
tomato
thin slices red onion
1 tsp Italian dressing
lettuce
(201 calories, 5 grams fat)

1) Spray non-stick griddle or skillet generously with butter-flavored spray.
2) Lay bread on a serving plate. Layer with cheese, tomato, onion, and Italian dressing.
3) Place another slice of bread on top of sandwich. Spray the top of the sandwich generously with butter-flavored spray.
4) Brown sandwiches over medium heat until golden brown. Turn over gently and brown the other side.

Your Workbook

Exercises, Questions, Tips, & Points to Ponder for Week 10 of Fight the Fat

The Bulletin Board

"The great composer does not set to work because he is inspired,
but becomes inspired because he is working."
—Ernest Newman

"Focus on remedies, not faults."
—Jack Nicklaus

"Every day old dogs learn new tricks."
—Alan Joseph

"When you stop learning, stop listening, stop looking,
and asking questions, then it is time to die."
—Lillian Smith

"People are like stained-glass windows. They sparkle and
shine when the sun is out, but when the darkness sets in,
their true beauty is revealed only if there is a light from within."
—Elizabeth Kübler-Ross

"Perseverance is not a long race. It is many short races, one after another."
—Walter Elliott

"In the long run you hit only what you aim at. Therefore, though you should fail
immediately, you had better aim at something high."
—Henry David Thoreau

Your Journal

List some of the NEW goals you are setting for your future! In deciding these, ask yourself:

1) What part of the program did I find most difficult or challenging?

2) What part of the program did I find easy to implement right away?

3) Who in my life do I see as being most helpful/supportive during this time of change?

4) How will I acknowledge or show my gratitude to that person/persons?

5) Who in my life do I see as being most difficult to deal with during this time of change?

6 What will be my strategy for dealing with that person/persons?

Healthy Habit for the Week

Calcium is essential for maintaining strong bones, but studies show that many Americans aren't complementing their calcium intake with vitamin D—and without vitamin D, the calcium cannot be absorbed as efficiently. Dairy food and eggs contain D, as do fortified cereals. But the sun is even better. Twenty minutes of soaking up the rays, three times a week on the face, hands, and arms will give you more than your required daily amount. So, take a walk *on the sunny side of the street.* But, remember not to overdo it!

Reward for the Week

In keeping with this week's theme of review, of incorporating new habits into your daily life, pick a reward from a previous week that you've *already* tried and enjoyed and repeat it again.

Can you see making this part of your weekly or daily pattern? Incorporating a reward into your life is a whole different ball game from trying it once. It's human nature to revert to *old* patterns—like a stream returning to its old course after the rains are over. No matter how much you've enjoyed something, you still have to fight *inertia*, past patterns and old habits to enable you to create a new lifestyle. This week's *repetition* is in itself a good habit, a good way to remember *I enjoyed that, and I deserve to have it become part of my life.*

Team Activity for the Week

Game time. Try an athletic event to perk up a meeting. Try tennis, for example, for a two-member team. Volleyball is also a good idea for two or more. Get on the court and give your new muscles a workout!

Even if your normal team activity is aerobics or walking or jogging, it will add an element of drama if you feel that you are *preparing* for some event like a race or (for those who don't like competition) an extra-long walk. Walking those ten miles to your friend's house will be a measure of how far you've come. It might be a one-time feat, but still it represents something the old you never would have dreamed of.

Julie, a Fight the Fat member, said, "I didn't realize what those twenty-minute walks did for me until my car broke down. It was cold and no one was coming along, so instead of just standing there getting more and more stressed out, I decided to walk to the garage about seven miles away. Half-way there someone I knew stopped to give me a lift—but what a difference that walk made in my mood. I wasn't even tired and could have walked the whole way. Talk about feeling on top of the world!"

Golden Rule for the Week

Never get up from the table feeling hungry, frustrated, irritable, and deprived! If you feel that you have to cheat a little to lift your mood, do it! An extra piece of fruit, or another serving of meat or fish or bread won't have significant consequences in terms of your weight loss. You can work them off when you are up to it. Feeling deprived or unhappy with your meal *can* have serious consequences. Think big picture. Think long-term.

Food of the Week

Technically they're an herb—the largest one around. But the real reasons *bananas* deserve a mention apart from the other fruits are that they:

- come in at a mere one hundred calories;
- are Rockefeller rich in potassium;
- are low in fat;
- may lower your risk-category for stroke and high blood pressure;
- are the basis for any good smoothie; and
- can be frozen when they start to get spotty and kept for a few weeks after that.

Gourmet author Susan Quick has recently written a book called *Go Bananas* that will give you new ideas about how to enjoy them. She lists 150 banana recipes ranging from curries to pancakes!

So, for a sweet treat that's rich in magnesium (a mineral that helps bones absorb calcium), and for an easily digested source of energy (athletes often reach for one for a quick surge of power), try imitating the monkeys for a change! Go ape over bananas!

Self-empowerment Exercise for the Week

There are many stories of people who have suffered poverty remaining fearful and insecure even after they've achieved wealth. The *reality* for them is somewhere back in the past. It's what they were used to—in a way it's what they were comfortable with. *Tomorrow it can all change back!* they lament, making everyone around them miserable with their frugality.

And the same is true when it comes to weight. It's just as hard to change the way we feel about our new selves as it was to change our bodies. "Members come up to me after the week ten meeting is over," says Bobbi Schell, Supervisor of Rehabilitation Outreach Services at Mercy. "Though they've done very well during the campaign—lost a lot of weight and toned up their bodies—they feel insecure now. *I'm scared!* they tell me.

I'm afraid that I'll wake up tomorrow morning the old me. I try to talk them out of their fears, but since it's not rational to begin with, arguments don't work. They have to change their self-image gradually, over time."

Self-image is a vital issue at this stage. As a person used to viewing yourself as sedentary and without willpower, you must learn to see yourself as active, fit, and in control. But if you're someone who has had a weight problem all their life, if your mother and father nagged you about it and made you feel terrible because of it, if they themselves had a weight problem, if you always had a wardrobe of fat, super-fat, and "tent" clothes, and if you have been on every weight loss program around, from Slim Fast to Atkins to the Scarsdale Torture—make that Diet—how are you supposed to suddenly feel comfortable in a bikini?

For starters, it's a good idea to surround yourself with photos of the new you. Everywhere. Second of all, spend some time every day, before work, in the evening, naked—absolutely nude—in front of the mirror. Get to know your body without shame.

Make lists of ways in which you have changed since joining Fight the Fat, and review them often. Jot down ways in which you can build on these changes. Throw out those old "fat" wardrobes and dress in ways that show off your new body shape. Most important of all, talk out your feelings with your teammate(s). There was an old saying, *Confession is good for the soul.* Well, there's a psychological basis for that as well as a religious one. Studies have shown that people who confide in others—as opposed to loners—are at a lower risk for a wide range of sicknesses and have a longer life expectancy as well. There's nothing more healing than friendship to help you overcome the pain of the past.

Stress Antidote for the Week

Simplify! Simplify! Simplify! This is even truer today than it was when Thoreau said it. Modern life seems to fill our days with endless details, endless clutter, and meaningless complications. Just lose your wallet and you'll realize to what extent we are entangled in a web of credit cards and cells phones and forms! When you live in a disorganized manner, that daily search for the car keys, that *overdue* notice from the bank or library, that *Where did I put it? Didn't I pay it?* syndrome can leave you with a pounding heart and a splitting headache.

From the basic rule of organization (always put things back in one place) to the complex art of dealing with your money and managing your time, there are excellent guides that will finally help you get your life in order. And you will feel better not dreading a bounced check notice as you sort through a mountain of junk mail! Deciding what—and who—comes first in your life will take the agony out of decisions and leave you with time for the things that really matter.

Progressive Relaxation

There are many different ways to skin the cat known as *progressive relaxation*. It's taught by yoga instructors, by physical therapists, and by psychologists who find that it helps the patient overcome inhibitions during their sessions.

As Dr. Andrew Weil says in *Natural Health, Natural Medicine,* "Progressive relaxation is a way of releasing tension in muscles...Most [instructors] begin by having you lie on your back in a comfortable position. Take a series of deep slow breaths and then focus your awareness of different part of the body, in turn becoming aware of any muscular tension and releasing it. One way to do this is to first tense a muscle deliberately and then relax it."

The key word here is "slow." If you rush through progressive relaxation as part of a busy schedule it won't work. You have to forget everything but the part of the body you are concentrating on.

Take the face; it's a good barometer of how you feel and the first step in getting rid of unwanted tension is to become aware of it. Is your tongue at the bottom of your mouth as it should be in a relaxed mood? Is your forehead smoothed or puckered up in concentration? Are your jaws clenched? Open the mouth wide (no forcing) and inhale. Exhale slowly as you close your mouth, lightly massaging the jaw muscles. Do you feel the difference? This is the kind of slow, steady examination that can be repeated up and down your body. Nirvana here I come!

Bibliography

Balch, Phyllis A., and James F. Balch, M.D. *Prescriptions for Dietary Wellness.* New York: Avery Penguin Putnam, 1998.

Benson, Herbert, M.D. *The Relaxation Response.* New York: Avon Books, 1974.

—*Beyond the Relaxation Response.* New York: Times Books, 1984.

Berg, Frances, M. *Children and Teens Afraid to Eat.* Hettinger, ND: Healthy Weight Journal, 2000.

Bortz, Walter, M.D. *Dare to Be 100.* New York: Fireside, 1996.

Borysenko, Joan. *Minding the Body, Mending the Mind.* Boston, MA: Addison-Wesley, 1994.

Carlson, Richard. *Don't Sweat the Small Stuff...and It's All Small Stuff.* New York: Hyperion, 1997.

Carnegie, Dale. *How to Win Friends and Influence People.* New York: Pocket Books, 1994.

"Carrot Soup." *Fitness Magazine* Nov. 2000.

"Citrus Chicken with Yogurt-Jalapeno Sauce." *Prevention Magazine* March 1996.

Colby, Anne. *Daily Meditations for Dieters.* Sacramento, CA: Citadel Press, 1994.

Connor, Sonja L., and William E. Connor, M.D. *The New American Diet Cookbook.* New York: Simon & Schuster, 1997.

Covey, Stephen R. *Daily Reflections for Highly Effective People.* New York: Fireside, 1994.

—*The 7 Habits of Highly Effective People.* New York: Fireside, 1990.

—*First Things First.* New York: Fireside, 1996.

—*Principle-Centered Leadership.* New York: Fireside, 1992.

Dreher, Henry. *Your Defense Against Cancer.* New York: HarperCollins, 1988.

Easwaran, Eknath. *Meditation.* Tomales, CA: Nilgiri Press, 1991.

Francina, Suza. *The New Yoga for People Over 50.* Deerfield Beach, FL: Health Communications, Inc., 1997.

Franz, Marion J. *Fast Food Facts*. Minnetonka, MN: Chronimed Publishing, 1994.

"Ginger, Green Apple, Sweet Onion and Coconut Salad." *Food & Wine* May 2001.

Gullo, Stephen P., M.D. *Thin Tastes Better*. New York: Dell Publishing, 1996.

Hansen, Vikki, and Shawn Goodman. *The 7 Secrets of Slim People*. New York: HarperCollins, 1999.

Henner, Marilu. *Total Health Makeover*. New York: ReganBooks, 1998.

Kaufman, Rosalie. *Yes You Can!* New York: Kensington Press, 1999.

Lanza, Louis. *Totally Dairy-Free Cooking*. New York: William Morrow, 2000.

Lasater, Judith. *Relax and Renew: Restful Yoga for Stressful Times*. Berkeley, CA: Rodmell Press, 1995.

"Lemongrass Chicken." *Food & Wine* May 2001.

LeShan, Lawrence. *How to Meditate*. New York: Little Brown & Co., 1999.

Radcliffe, Rebecca R. *Enlightened Eating*. Ease Publications and Resources, 1996. (800) 470-GROW (4769).

Rossman, Martin L., M.D., *Healing Yourself*. Cape Coral, FL: Awareness Press, 1987.

Schaef, Anne Wilson. *Meditations for Women Who Do Too Much*. San Francisco: HarperCollins, 1996.

Shapiro, Howard M.D. *Dr. Shapiro's Picture Perfect Weight Loss*. Emmaus, PA: Rodale Press, 2000.

Shoshanna, Brenda, Ph.D. *Zen Miracles*. New York: John Wiley, 2002.

—*Why Men Leave*. New York: Perigree, 1999.

—*What He Can't Tell You...and Needs to Say*. New York: Perigree, 2001.

Simonton, O. Carl, M.D., Matthew Simonton, and James Creighton. *Getting Well Again*. New York: Bantam, 1992.

Smith, M.J. *All-American Low-fat and No-fat Meals in Minutes*. New York: John Wiley & Sons, 1997.

—*60 Days of Low-fat, Low-cost Meals in Minutes*. New York: John Wiley & Sons, 1998.

—*Daily Bread*. New York: John Wiley & Sons, 1997.

"Southwestern Barley." *Vegetarian Times* May 2001.

Stoll, Andrew, M.D. *The Omega-3 Connection.* New York: Free Press, 2001.

Sweetgall, Robert, and R. Whiteley, and Robert Neeves, Ph.D. *Walking Off Weight.* New York: The Lyons Press, 2001.

Weil, Andrew, M.D. *Natural Health, Natural Medicine.* Boston, MA: Houghton-Mifflin, 1998.

Wolff, Richard. *Big Fat Lies about Exercise and Fat Loss.* Elgin, IL: Wolff Health and Fitness Corporation, 1998.

—*Big Fat Lies about the Food You Eat.* Elgin, IL: Wolff Health and Fitness Corporation, 2001.

—*The New Diet Book Disaster.* Elgin, IL: Wolff Health and Fitness Corporation, 2000.

—*The Top 10 Fat Loss Plans of 1999.* Elgin, IL: Wolff Health and Fitness Corporation, 1999.

—*HMR Calorie System Checkbook.* Boston, MA: Health Management Resources Corporation, 2000.

—*HMR Calorie System Book.* Boston, MA: Health Management Resources Corporation, 1993.

Internet Sites, Useful Phone Numbers, and Useful Information

Eating plans tailored to your needs: www.ediets.com

Another tool that is not as comprehensive as ediets, but is still valuable and free: mealsforyou.com

For healthy suggestions and medical news: www.mayo clinic.com

Helpful meditations and advice on a wide range of issues by Dr. Brenda Shoshanna, the relationship expert: www.Brendashoshanna.com

For inspiring stories about people who have lived long, long healthy and rich lives: http://www.npr.org/programs/morning/100years.html

American Massage Therapy Association: www.amtamassage.org
(888) 843-2682

Food and fitness information: www.foodfit.com

The National Association for Health & Fitness, a non-profit organization made up of state councils to promote physical activity nationwide: www.healthyweightnetwork.com

Yoga Journal: www.yogajournal.com

Audobon Society: www.audobon.org/bird/birdathon

American Hiking Society: (301) 565-6704

Nutrition Action Health Letter
Center For Science in the Public Interest
1875 Connecticut Avenue, N.W., Suite 300
Washington, DC 20009-5728

Yoga Journal's Yoga Teachers Directory
Yoga Journal's Book and Tape Source
2054 University Avenue
Berkeley, CA 94704
www.yogajournal.com

Speakers

If your local Fight the Fat campaign ends up getting large enough so that you have the resources to invite speakers, here are a few recommendations to start you off. The following people have addressed Dyersville Fight the Fat meetings and have achieved excellent results:

Connie Bandy Hodge is a certified personal trainer, body builder, and motivational speaker. hodgecb@aol.com

Connie's motivational seminars on fitness aren't just talk. She's competed in power lifting, body building, and adventure racing, and she's participated, taught, and coached at the college level. Juggling her commitment to her personal fitness, her family of four, and her fitness business gives her insights into the challenges everyone experiences in getting and staying fit. Connie energetically and enthusiastically promotes self-respect and lifetime wellness.

Rob Bell spreads his motivational humor through Focus Presentations. robertbell@rocketmail.com

It's more fun to be excellent than mediocre, and that's a choice we all can make. Rob encourages conscious choices to appreciate the good things in our lives, to take responsibility for building positive relationships, to present a positive image to the world, and to honor others. Rob uses humor and anecdotes to engage his audience, and shares practical wisdom from his life experience.

Sandra A. Schuette is a lifestyles counselor in weight and stress management. Living Slim, Inc. dansandy@chorus.net

Sandy stresses that people's thoughts dictate their experience and that we have to change our thoughts in the weight loss process. Until our thinking is in alignment with healthy eating and exercise, the struggle will continue and weight will yo-yo up and down. In her interactive workshops, Sandy outlines specific techniques to help us change our way of thinking over time so that healthy habits will develop naturally from within. Her approach teaches people how to become their own coach rather than their own critic. Once thoughts are permanently changed, motivation and high self-esteem replace hopelessness.

Matt Taylor, MPT, RYT, is a physical therapist experienced in orthopedic and sports physical therapy. He is also a registered advanced level yoga therapist. matt@yogatherapy.com

Matt discusses the holistic approach to body weight management, exploring the interrelationship of breath, emotions, and physical movement. With candor and humor, he invites his audience to sample basic yoga while he balances theory with experience, and science with metaphor. His gift for translating the allegorical language of Eastern exercise systems into Western scientific terminology (and plain English!) gives participants the opportunity to enhance their health with these ancient traditions.